Why on Earth Do I Feel This Way?

*Understanding Anxiety and
Mental Health through Control Theory*

JOLENE ARASZ, Psy.D.

PAGE PUBLISHING, INC.
Conneaut Lake, PA

First originally published by Page Publishing 2020

This book is for educational purposes. It is not to replace or substitute any treatment by a doctor or other mental health-care provider.

ISBN 978-1-6624-1391-9 (pbk)
ISBN 978-1-6624-3267-5 (hc)
ISBN 978-1-6624-1392-6 (digital)

Printed in the United States of America

To be yourself in a world that is constantly trying to make you something else is the greatest accomplishment.

—Ralph Waldo Emerson

Contents

Introduction

On a summer afternoon, a mother brought her nineteen-year-old son to my office, complaining of him always being angry and yelling at her. Her son was silent throughout much of the session, slouching back in the chair, crossing his arms, looking at the floor, and rolling his eyes every time his mother spoke. I obviously knew he did not want to be sitting in my office. I was the third therapist to whom his mother had brought him. According to him, therapy was pointless. He had never benefited from it before and assumed I was going to be the same as every other therapist with whom he had worked. He didn't see any point in being there. As his mother continued to talk and describe his behavior, and not in the most supportive way, the dynamic between them materialized. I had to interrupt their exchange of words and started to describe my treatment approach. I didn't ask the son any questions during the intake. I knew he was not interested in talking, and I wasn't going to push him in our first meeting. However, I was hoping he would listen to what I had to say.

I described how my focus with my clients is anxiety based. I explained that every single person has anxiety, but it looks different from one person to the next. I described what anxiety is and that anxiety is actually rooted in feeling a lack of control. When we don't have the level of control we need or want, our anxiety automatically intensifies. When the anxiety increases, that is where we see the behaviors. Every single one of us reacts to anxiety in our own way, whether it's something big or something small. That's what hooked him. His head popped up when I described the way in which control, or lack thereof, is at the root of our anxiety. I normalized it. I

7

also caught the mother's attention. I then explained to him what we would work on to tackle that anxiety and put the control back into his hands. My client continued to come back to therapy every week until he went back to college, and by that time, he felt a whole other level of control that he never knew he could have.

Why on Earth Do I Feel This Way? aims to provide a basic understanding of anxiety and its impact on our daily lives. I'm writing this in hopes that I can raise awareness about and normalize anxiety and mental health. As a psychologist, my primary focus is helping my clients understand, become more aware of, and get control of their anxiety. *Control theory* addresses just that. Anxiety is ubiquitous, underrecognized, and undertreated under the current paradigms. Control theory offers a way to look at anxiety differently, to recognize its many forms, and to focus on certain aspects of anxiety that people can identify and gain control over.

The reason I feel it is so important for us to understand anxiety is that anxiety is at the root of everything with which we deal on a daily basis. The topic of anxiety is such an important topic for me. I have found, through years of practice, that anxiety is severely misunderstood, yet every single person experiences it. The problem is that most people are not necessarily aware that they are experiencing anxiety on a daily basis and easily misinterpret what they experience on a physical, mental, and emotional level.

While I hope to provide my readers with a better (or more accurate) understanding of anxiety, I also hope to increase their understanding of how to appropriately and effectively control their anxiety. I want my readers to walk away from this book having a more in-depth understanding of where in the world anxiety comes from, as well as the ability to utilize cognitive objectives to help decrease or prevent the use of maladaptive behaviors as a way to alleviate anxiety in a given moment.

The information provided in this book on anxiety and control theory can be utilized by various demographics. The objectives can be used by adolescents, adults, parents (and parents applying these tools for younger-age children), teachers, and other school personnel. My ultimate vision is for schools to require that mental health education be integrated as part of the mainstream curriculum, just as science, history, math, English, and other languages are. Until then, if we can start to implement these strategies in our schools, whether it be in elementary, middle school, high school, or even college settings, we can help students understand their anxiety in a way that helps facilitate the following areas: improving academic performance, stabilizing social relationships, prioritizing their individual needs and focusing on themselves in a healthy way, improving communication and interpersonal skills, setting clear and appropriate boundaries with others as well as for themselves, and learning how to take accountability for their own choices and responsibilities and how to hold others accountable. Control theory and the cognitive objectives presented in this book aim to not only help us understand anxiety and its causes but also to help in preventing or decreasing maladaptive behaviors, such as drinking, substance use, self-injurious behaviors, and violence.

Lastly, school violence and gun control have been discussed and debated at length throughout our country; however, there has not been a consistent approach to mediating these issues. Gun control will continue to be debated. Unfortunately, no matter what the law states, we will continue to see escalated violence unless we get to the root of the matter. Violence is something we can work toward decreasing. In order to do this, we need to learn what causes us to think about and engage in such behaviors. If we can understand what is precipitating these thoughts, we can learn healthier, more appropriate ways to exercise control, rather than resort to aggressive and violent behaviors.

The vision of this book is to better equip students as well as adults to take on the challenges of modern society's stressors. Grounded in the proven methods of cognitive-behavioral theory, control theory will help students learn how to exercise control in healthy and appropriate ways in all aspects of their lives, thus helping prevent more severe symptoms or other potential mental health disorders, as well as preventing or decreasing maladaptive behaviors. We can all have a healthy level of control in our lives, but we need to put some effort into learning about our anxiety and take accountability for our choices and actions. We have the power to gain healthy control, and when we do, we can make a big difference not only for ourselves but also in the world around us. This theory can be applied for all ages.

PART 1

Anxiety Background

How Has Anxiety Traditionally Been Defined?

In order to understand what anxiety is, particularly through control theory, we first need to understand how anxiety is currently defined. According to the *Diagnostic and Statistical Manual of Mental Disorders, Fifth Edition: DSM-5* (American Psychiatric Association 2013), *anxiety* is defined as an "anticipation of a future threat." Fear is also a component of anxiety, where the *DSM-5* defines *fear* as the "emotional response to a real or perceived imminent threat."

The *DSM-5* presents several differential diagnoses of anxiety disorders, including generalized anxiety disorder, social anxiety, phobias, separation anxiety, selective mutism, and panic disorder. There is not much differentiation among these anxiety disorders, other than the actual object or circumstance that triggers the anxiety. In order for anxiety to reach a clinical, diagnosable level, the *DSM* states that a person's daily functioning has been compromised (based on their set of symptoms) for a certain period of time (depending on age), and the anxiety is not attributed to the physiological effects of a substance or medication or due to another medical condition and is not better explained by another mental disorder. Here is where control theory takes a different approach. As we get into control theory, we will not just be focusing on anxiety as it reaches the level of becoming a disorder; rather, we will be looking at how typical anxiety plays a role in our day-to-day lives that is often overlooked or unrecognized. Control theory can be applied even when we aren't experiencing extremely high levels of anxiety for basic anxiety that we may experience on a daily basis. Unfortunately, anxiety can be ubiquitous and misunderstood, which makes us vulnerable to not recognizing or appropriately treating our anxiety. Control theory has a much broader approach to understanding anxiety and does not put as much emphasis on treating the specific symptoms that are manifested as a result of anxiety. Control theory focuses on the underlying cause and provides an educational approach to helping people understand why they are feeling anxious in the first place.

Conventional Treatments and Theories

There have been a few common theories and treatment approaches to help manage anxiety as well as other disorders. One of the most common and empirically supported treatment approaches is that of cognitive behavioral therapy (CBT). Other treatment approaches that have been helpful for managing anxiety include mindfulness, dialectical behavior therapy (DBT), and eye movement desensitization and reprocessing (EMDR). Mindfulness focuses on feeling grounded in the present moment. DBT focuses on teaching emotional regulation or how to better manage or control your emotions, and EMDR focuses on alleviating stress resulting from trauma or disturbing life experiences. All these approaches are beneficial, but even these approaches have a common theme that isn't outwardly addressed in the theoretical explanations. That theme is control. Control theory can be utilized alongside these theoretical approaches to help people understand why each of these theories can be successful. Each approach has its own objectives and specific goals. However, if we break down the objectives and recognize the end goals, each theory provides tools to help people increase their own personal sense of control. Control theory provides a more general overall picture of how our focus on control can be applied across various life experiences.

Although control theory has a different approach to understanding and managing anxiety than other, more conventional theories, much of my clinical work is based on the teachings of Judith Beck, who uses cognitive theory, stemming from the work of Aaron Beck. Both Aaron and Judith Beck have been and continue to be highly regarded as being among the most prominent psychologists in the field of cognitive therapy. Aaron Beck developed cognitive therapy in the 1960s. Cognitive therapy aims to be "a structured, short-term, present-oriented psychotherapy for depression, directed toward solving current problems and modifying dysfunctional thinking and behavior" (Beck [1964] 1995). Cognitive therapy is specifically focused on identifying dysfunctional thoughts and replacing these thoughts with alternative, positive thoughts. The cognitive model presents several principles that guide the focus of the work. Some of the cognitive principles include assessing one's thinking in the current moment, assessing problematic behaviors that result from distorted thoughts, identifying precipitating factors that influence a person's thought process, and identifying developmental events that influence a person's thought process and thought patterns. Cognitive therapy is goal oriented and problem focused and aims to be educational and prevent relapse. Cognitive theory teaches people how to identify, evaluate, and respond to their dysfunctional thoughts (Beck 1995).

There are many common objectives in control theory and cognitive theory, including being initially present oriented, identifying precipitating factors to anxiety, and identifying the thoughts and beliefs that trigger anxiety and the behaviors that result from that anxiety. They also both explore a person's developmental history, which may be influencing the way in which they interpret information. Both theories are educational in nature and aim to be preventive approaches to managing mental health issues and to managing anxiety more effectively in the future.

Where control theory differs from Judith Beck's cognitive theory is that Beck focuses on the importance of distinguishing between emotions and thought analysis, while control theory presents a much broader description of anxiety. Control theory views any negative emotion as a symptom of anxiety and focuses on a lack of control as the stimulus for anxiety. For example, Beck states that feeling anxious is different than feeling sad. Control theory views any negative emotion as a way in which anxiety is manifested. According to control theory, each emotion is unique but is also a way of communicating that something doesn't feel right, and the individual doesn't have the level of control they need in that moment. Cognitive theory doesn't address control, or lack thereof, as being a cause for anxiety.

Another way to distinguish control theory from cognitive theory is that control theory identifies the underlying theme of beliefs or the root cause of anxiety that sets the stage for our anxiety as we continue through development and into adulthood, while cognitive theory analyzes each belief independently. The main objective of control theory is to teach others to shift control back into their own hands, which decreases their anxiety and increases their overall personal sense of control over themselves and the circumstances that triggered anxiety for them.

Control theory also differs from another psychological concept, *locus of control*. Locus of control refers to how a person views their self. An internal locus of control means someone feels their personal efforts and abilities are the reason they are successful. An external locus of control means that a person perceives their successes as being due to external factors or luck. According to this theory, those who have an external locus of control are less likely to put forth significant effort to achieve something. They view their success as depending on circumstances, almost feeling as though they have limited to no control over the outcome. A person with an internal locus of control is assumed to be more achievement driven. Control theory does not view a person's sense of control to be one or the other. Rather, control theory works on teaching people to accept the things over which they don't have control and then shift their focus to those things that are within their control and identify what their other options are, using a problem-solving approach.

Anxiety typically doesn't just show up in only one aspect of our lives. Anxiety plays a role in our daily lives, which is why it is highly misunderstood, misdiagnosed, and mistreated. Cognitive theory does provide ways in which we can identify our anxious thoughts and replace them with more positive thoughts. However, as helpful as cognitive theory has been, there is still a missing link in terms of understanding the origins of anxiety.

Medication

Medication can be a controversial subject. I have been practicing CBT for several years, and it has been very rare for me to recommend my clients for medication in addition to therapy when specifically practicing CBT. The reason I seldom recommend my clients for medication is that I feel CBT and control theory are very successful based on the amount of progress I see in my clients within a short period of time. I tend to see progress with my clients very early in their treatment if they choose to apply the clinical work they are learning in therapy in their daily lives. The more effort and practice my clients put into managing their anxiety, the more progress I see, and the faster I see it.

If I see progress with a client, I interpret that as the client better understanding their anxiety and starting to practice skills that allow them to increase their self-reliance rather than depending on someone or something else to help them feel better. When they start to see evidence that they have the power to decrease their anxiety because of the steps they are taking, not only do their overall sense of control increase and their baseline average daily level of anxiety decrease, but their self-confidence and happiness increase as well.

Although it's rare that I recommend that my clients take medication, I am not completely opposed to using it. When I have been working with a client for a few sessions and have some time to assess their anxiety and how they have been managing it over a few weeks' time, I am able to gather enough information to see how intense their anxiety is on a day-to-day and week-to-week-basis. I will also be able to assess if my client is willing or even able to do the clinical work if their anxiety is extremely high. Medication is to be used to help the client's anxiety decrease a couple of notches on the scale to the point where they can focus a little more clearly, have better concentration, and are able to think through the clinical steps that are needed to decrease their anxiety. Medication is not supposed to take away anxiety or depression. It is not supposed to numb the client. It is supposed to help alleviate the anxiety to the point where they are then able to do the clinical work to bring their anxiety down to a more manageable level on a day-to-day basis.

Unfortunately, it is very rare that I have a client who has either been on medication or goes on medication who is taught how to use their medication appropriately by the prescribing doctor. Medication for anxiety (or depression or any other mental health symptoms) should be used in conjunction with therapy. When clients are not utilizing therapy while taking medication to manage mental health symptoms, they are not increasing the level of awareness of their anxiety. They are becoming more dependent on the medication to help them feel better, often expecting the medication to take all their symptoms away, and are not understanding why they are feeling anxious (or depressed) in the first place. They are not learning where their anxiety originates or how their thought patterns are triggering their anxiety. They are not becoming educated about their anxiety and, therefore, are not increasing their skills to manage their anxiety or depression. They are dependent on a foreign substance to manage their symptoms.

PART 2

New Practice: Control Theory

What Is Control Theory, and How Is It Different from Previous Theories?

Throughout the course of my work over the past seventeen years, I have been able to develop an alternative theory of how to understand anxiety, which I refer to as control theory. Control theory is a new theoretical approach to understanding what anxiety is and where it originates and provides ways in which we can manage anxiety by focusing on our personal sense of control. Control theory is based on the notion that anxiety develops when we are experiencing a lack of personal control. When we don't have the level of control that we need or want, our anxiety increases. It provides a more general understanding of anxiety and a thematic approach to applying control theory in all aspects of life.

Many theoretical approaches to managing mental health are based on symptoms that, together, present as a disorder and focus on the diagnosis or class of symptoms. Control theory specifically focuses on anxiety and anxiety management because anxiety is at the root of any mental health disorder. By tackling the root cause of a disorder and learning how to control the underlying anxiety, we are able to minimize, decrease, or prevent the development of more severe symptoms that may then be categorized as another mental health disorder. Anxiety is ubiquitous, underrecognized, and undertreated under the current theoretical and treatment paradigms. Control theory offers a way to look at anxiety differently, to recognize its many forms, and to focus on certain aspects of anxiety that people can identify and gain control over.

What Is Anxiety According to Control Theory?

So how does control theory define anxiety? According to control theory, anxiety is triggered when we experience a lack of sense of control. This may seem like a broad and vague description of anxiety. It is. That's part of why control theory is unique. Control theory uses *anxiety* as a very general term. Control theory views anxiety as any uncomfortable feeling that we experience. This includes feeling sad, angry, irritable, nervous, scared, etc. Any uncomfortable feeling—that's anxiety. It's our body's natural way of saying, "Something isn't right here! I don't feel like my normal self." It's that natural fight-or-flight response when we don't feel we have the level of control we need or want in a particular situation. You may be wondering, How is sadness anxiety? If you think about a time when you have felt sad, did you feel like you had control over the circumstances that made you feel sad? Chances are you were feeling sad because a situation was not going in a way in which you chose, and you felt your control was limited in some capacity.

Although anxiety has primarily served as a survival mechanism for all species, it has evolved for humans in such a way that it no longer serves our best self-interest. Our problem-solving abilities and social-emotional functioning are compromised as a result. I will discuss in greater detail how these compromises are manifested later in the book.

Let's compare control theory's definition of *anxiety* to the description of *anxiety* in the *DSM-5*. As previously mentioned, the

DSM emphasizes anxiety based on excessive fear, stating that "fear is the emotional response to a real or perceived imminent threat." Fear differs from anxiety, according to the *DSM*: "Anxiety is anticipation of future threat." The *DSM* also lists panic attacks as a fear response.

Now let's think about fear and anxiety coming from the perspective of control theory. When we think about experiencing or perceiving a threat, what happens to our sense of control? It drops. If we are feeling threatened, we are not going to feel like we have control over what is happening to us or around us. If we do feel we have a greater sense of control, then our anxiety won't feel overwhelming, and we won't feel so threatened. The common thread that shows up in every case of anxiety is not a fear response; it's really a lack of feeling in control. Even if fear is strictly an emotional response, as the *DSM* states, that fear is still triggered when we don't have the control we need in that moment. When we anticipate something that triggers our anxiety, again, we are feeling a lack of control if we are anticipating a negative event.

When we perceive or anticipate an imminent or future threat, we don't feel we have a strong sense of control. If we are feeling sad, angry, annoyed, etc., then we are likely not feeling the level of control we would like; therefore, our anxiety (negative feeling) becomes stronger. When something doesn't go the way we planned, we don't feel we have the level of control that we want or need. When we don't get what we want, we feel a loss of control, resulting in frustration, anger, irritability, etc. When we undergo any kind of change or transition, we don't always have the level of control that we want or with which we would feel comfortable because we can't predict how the events will transpire. If we know exactly how our life transitions will play out or can predict how changes or events will transpire, knowing exactly what to expect, then we will experience a higher level of control, which will naturally keep our level of anxiety low.

These are only a few examples of how the lack of a sense of control triggers a higher level of anxiety. I will go into further detail of how anxiety and control (or lack thereof) are present in other critical areas of our lives. First, let's get a better understanding of what the anxiety scale represents.

How Do We Better Recognize Anxiety? Applying the Anxiety Scale

To make anxiety more tangible, I will be using a numerical scale as a reference throughout the reading to demonstrate ways in which anxiety plays a role in various areas of our lives. The higher we are on the scale, the lower our sense of control or ability to personally affect a given outcome in a particular situation or circumstance will be. The numerical scale ranges from 0 to 10, where 10 represents the most intense level of anxiety. When our anxiety is high, we are actually experiencing low levels of control. This is the focus of our work: control. As we learn about anxiety, I will be focusing on the ways in which anxiety is rooted in experiencing a lack of control.

Using the anxiety scale can help us gain a better sense of awareness of how our anxiety is affecting us from moment to moment. It provides a visual tool to help us gauge the level of intensity of anxiety in the moment. Again, when our sense of anxiety is higher on the scale, it is due to our low sense of control. Below is a brief description of what anxiety levels may feel like on the scale from 0 to 10:

Anxiety Scale

10 — Completely overwhelmed. I definitely can't focus or concentrate. I'm experiencing intense symptoms of anxiety: somatic symptoms, heart palpitations, anxiety, and panic attacks. I don't know what to do to calm myself down. I feel like I can't do anything without my anxiety controlling me and getting in the way.

8–9 — Overwhelming anxiety or stress. I'm having a very difficult time focusing and concentrating. I can be short-tempered and easily reactive toward others. It feels like I spend all my day's energy thinking about my anxiety or what makes me feel anxious.

7 — Feeling more overwhelmed. Now I don't even want to deal with the stressor. I want to be left alone and not talk about or deal with the issue at hand. Even though I may not want to talk about the issue at hand, I am still able to talk about it.

6 — Stress is increasing. I don't feel I have as much control as I would like, but maybe if I talk to someone about it, I can figure out what to do.

5 — Anxiety is there, and I'm aware of it, but I am able to manage it. I don't spend my day focusing on my anxiety. My anxiety is manageable and doesn't really cause my family or anyone else a big problem.

4 — Starting to feel anxious. Possibly anticipating something I don't want to deal with, but I'm not in the midst of the potential stressor.

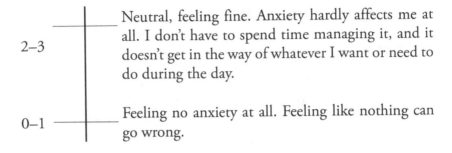

2–3 — Neutral, feeling fine. Anxiety hardly affects me at all. I don't have to spend time managing it, and it doesn't get in the way of whatever I want or need to do during the day.

0–1 — Feeling no anxiety at all. Feeling like nothing can go wrong.

By applying the scale and giving ourselves a number we can identify when experiencing stress or anxiety, we are able to increase our emotional awareness. By using the scale, we can start to get a general understanding of our average level of anxiety on a daily basis. We become more aware of how much our anxiety may vacillate from day-to-day or even throughout the day. We can start to see how our anxiety increases as our sense of control decreases. Our personal awareness of our anxiety increases. In order to work toward gaining control over our anxiety, we need to increase our sense of awareness regarding our uncomfortable emotions. We will continue to explore how our thought process plays a role in the fluctuation of our anxiety and control throughout the reading.

How Anxiety Can Be Manifested

Anxiety can be manifested in countless ways, including emotional dysregulation and physical or somatic (bodily) symptoms. Anxiety can be manifested emotionally (through anger, irritability, nervousness, sadness, and any other uncomfortable feeling), behaviorally (through impulsivity, aggression, shutting down, etc.), and somatically (through headaches, shakiness, sweating, gastrointestinal problems, and other physical ailments, or through feeling restless, feeling on edge, being fatigued, experiencing sleep disturbance, having difficulty concentrating or having one's mind going blank, having muscle tension, worrying, having intrusive thoughts, etc.). It is very common for people who experience heightened levels of anxiety to develop gastrointestinal issues, including general abdominal pain, nausea, vomiting, irritable bowel syndrome (IBS), colitis, constipation, etc. Gastrointestinal problems are common in children and adults because the gut houses huge concentrations of nerves—almost as many as the brain. Our gut is actually considered to be our second brain because of how concentrated it is with nerves. These nerves react to stress just like our brain reacts. When these nerves are continuously reacting to stress, we are more prone to developing other symptoms in our gut.

Anxiety can also be masked as different disorders. Anxiety can present itself in numerous ways. A panic attack can often feel as though you are having a heart attack. Gastrointestinal issues also mask anxiety but are frequently diagnosed as other medical disorders. Although there are separate classifications of symptoms that make up a specific disorder, we need to look beyond strictly the physical and behavioral symptoms.

The first thing we need to assess is a person's anxiety. When clients have previously been diagnosed with a disorder based on a handful of symptoms, I always start my work with them (after gathering background information and family and treatment history), by providing an educational approach to explain anxiety and then assess their own anxiety. When I focus on understanding their anxiety as well as where it's rooted, we can then move forward with utilizing clinical tools to manage their anxiety moving forward. As we gain more control over the anxiety, the symptoms that we're providing diagnostic criteria for another disorder start to subside. It's not that these symptoms are not real (they are very real and can be excruciatingly painful), but we need to look at the underlying causes of these disorders and not just take the symptoms at face value.

When a client experiences symptoms of various mental health disorders, including bipolar disorder, obsessive-compulsive disorders, or even symptoms of psychosis, these symptoms are oftentimes triggered when the client is under high stress or high anxiety. The symptoms are a reaction or a defense mechanism when the client is feeling so overwhelmed that they lose their personal sense of control. I've also had clients tell me that they never felt like they didn't have control, but after learning about what healthy control over their anxiety feels like, they recognize that the "control" they thought they had before was more of a false sense of control and their body's way of reacting to anxiety or stress in maladaptive ways, though they did not recognize this at the time.

It can be comforting for some people to continuously engage in compulsive behaviors, helping them feel like they have a sense of control over something in the moment, and that behavior and obsession help them avoid focusing on or dealing with the primary stressor. Psychotic symptoms, as well as dissociation, can also bring a sense of relief for people when they feel completely overwhelmed with what is happening in their life in the moment; they can check out when they are feeling highly overwhelmed and it's too much to cognitively and emotionally process what they are experiencing in the moment. I'm not trying to say that anxiety is the only cause of other disorders or symptoms, such as psychosis, but these symptoms can be more easily triggered or escalated under stress or when anxiety is particularly high. Throughout my work, I have seen a consistent pattern when clients experience severe levels of anxiety. They are highly vulnerable to experiencing a wide range of symptoms.

When does anxiety become such a problem that it is considered to be a disorder? According to the *DSM-5*, anxiety becomes a disorder when it *persists beyond developmentally appropriate periods*. This means that the anxiety has been experienced for an extended period of time (typically six months or more, according to the *DSM-5* diagnostic criteria, but it may be less for children). Although every single person has anxiety, and it is beneficial at appropriate times, it does not mean that everyone meets the clinical criteria for a disorder.

However, just because not everyone meets the diagnostic criteria for an anxiety disorder does not mean that we shouldn't pay attention to or understand our own anxiety. In fact, if we learn more about our anxiety, pay more attention to the role it plays in our lives, and understand ways in which we can control it, we will be more likely to help prevent ourselves from reaching a diagnosable level of anxiety or other potential mental health issues. We will also be less likely to engage in maladaptive or unhealthy behaviors in a misguided effort to alleviate our anxiety. I will address how to use control theory as a preventive tool for maladaptive behaviors throughout the reading.

Although our anxiety can impede our functioning at times, it can also be very useful in certain situations. It can keep us vigilant when we are in dangerous situations, which is the primary purpose of anxiety. It's our warning signal when we are in danger or in an unsafe situation. It can also motivate us to get things done or work hard to achieve something, such as a job promotion or school success. This defense mechanism, a healthy anxiety, does indeed serve an important purpose, and we want to utilize this anxiety in healthy and productive ways. However, when anxiety starts to interfere with our ability to focus on other priorities and affects our level of performance on a consistent basis, then we need to recognize the extent to which our anxiety has become unhealthy and is interfering with our daily lives. We want to utilize our anxiety to the degree that it is useful while also working to control it as best we can when it impedes our functioning.

Understanding anxiety happens in many parts. We need to learn where our anxiety originates, what further triggers our anxiety, what it looks like for us independent of others, and how can we control it so we can direct our focus where it needs to be, bringing our anxiety levels down and increasing our sense of control.

Where Anxiety Begins: Core Beliefs and Automatic Thoughts

One aspect of Judith Beck's work that I have incorporated into my own practice is identifying automatic thoughts. *Automatic thoughts* are defined by Judith Beck as "the actual words or images that go through a person's mind, are situation specific, and may be considered the most superficial level of cognition" (Beck 2005, 16). According to Judith Beck, these automatic thoughts are based on our core beliefs, which we cultivate throughout our development, particularly in the earlier stages.

Core beliefs

Judith Beck's theory of core beliefs lay the foundation for understanding much of our automatic thoughts. According to Judith Beck, these core beliefs are global (not situation specific), rigid (very difficult to change), and overgeneralized. These are beliefs that we internalize when we are young and represent how we then perceive ourselves as individuals. One example of how core beliefs are developed is through a child's learning experience. Depending on whether a child has a positive or negative experience at a certain time or event of their life, that experience will influence how that child interprets their own sense of self, based on how successful they felt they were in managing that event.

Core beliefs can also develop based on how we interpret information or feedback from others. These experiences form core beliefs that we can potentially maintain throughout much of our lives and may not be correct, which influences our own self-esteem or sense of self-worth. When we have negative experiences, it is easy for us to interpret these experiences in a way that has a negative impact on our sense of self. We often assume we are at fault. We start to have negative thoughts about ourselves, feeling as though we are not good enough or are a failure. We believe these thoughts are true, and we internalize them as part of who we believe we are as a person, forming a negative sense of self.

Aaron Beck (1964) distinguishes between two different types of core beliefs: beliefs about ourselves and beliefs about others. I have found in my own practice that both of these types of core beliefs are equally common. A core belief that we may have about others can also stem from our early childhood experiences. We may believe that no one is trustworthy or that other people will hurt us. Aaron Beck refers to these core beliefs about others as *generalizations*. We need to work on understanding the context of these beliefs and identify if these thoughts are valid or not, based on supporting evidence. These core beliefs are likely to have repeatedly influenced our perceptions throughout our lives, so we can identify a pattern of when these core beliefs trigger our automatic thoughts, triggering our anxiety.

For example, if a child is abused at a young age, they are not likely to understand why the abuse is happening but can very easily start assuming that they deserve to be hurt because they did something wrong, they are not worthy of love and affection, they aren't good enough in some capacity, etc. These are core beliefs that quickly develop based on a child's early experience. As the child gets older, they may assume that others perceive them the same way, so any experience that reminds them of having been abused will trigger the same thoughts, which triggers their anxiety. They will often assume that they are not good enough, or they may think they deserve to be mistreated by others. Our negative core beliefs also directly affect our self-esteem and sense of self. I will address self-esteem in greater detail in the next chapter.

Additionally, someone who has a history of being abused may assume throughout their life that others (especially others who hold a similar relationship or dynamic as the child had with their abuser) will also abuse them. They may be constantly anticipating how others will react to them or treat them. They generalize their core belief that they can't trust people if they get too close to them or if they allow themselves to be vulnerable with another person.

Another example of developing core beliefs is when a young child experiences a loss in the sense of abandonment. If a child is placed in the care of others who were not their initial caretaker, especially after having already established a firm attachment with their initial caregiver, the child may then anticipate being abandoned by other caretakers or by others with whom they try to establish a relationship throughout their development and adulthood. Children who are adopted or spend time in foster care often struggle to allow themselves to fully engage in a relationship with a caretaker or other relationship, in fear of losing that significant person. It is common for a child who has not had the same caretakers their whole life, even as they continue to get older, to assume that they will be abandoned by others. They are likely to have a difficult time allowing themselves to fully engage in a relationship (romantic, friendship, or otherwise) without anticipating that the other person will leave them.

Even deeply ingrained core beliefs, however, are not necessarily true. Aaron Beck thought it was important to educate people about this—even when someone feels very strongly about something, it may be a false belief. Their experience is always valid, but they may be helped by learning to look at the concrete evidence for or against their automatic thoughts. We need to practice looking at the concrete evidence that may or may not support the automatic thoughts in a more logical way, without discounting how a person felt or feels. When we are able to identify examples of when someone experienced an event when there was evidence to prove that their core beliefs or automatic thoughts were not true, we can then work to modify core beliefs and automatic thoughts.

Automatic thoughts

Our negative core beliefs develop as we internalize negative thoughts or assumptions. Our negative core beliefs make us vulnerable to experiencing anxiety and a limited sense of control. We are more apt to assume negative things in vulnerable situations. In order to identify automatic thoughts, it is important to take inventory of what is happening in the moment we start to feel any anxiety. Judith Beck stresses that when our mood changes, we should ask ourselves what we are thinking about in that moment. If we are not able to identify the automatic thoughts that are triggering our anxiety outright, we should do an inventory of the situation: *Where am I? What is happening? Who am I with?* We should continue to question our automatic thoughts by asking, *What am I anticipating? What am I afraid of happening? What is my biggest concern or fear?*

These assumptions or anticipatory thoughts are the root cause that triggers our anxiety. We assume we are helpless; therefore, we minimize our sense of control. When we assume something negative, we believe the assumption to be true, and one automatic thought or assumption will trigger another and another and another, and soon, we are thinking about the worst-case scenario. We become consumed by these thoughts, prompting our helplessness or fears of impending disaster, and believe that these automatic thoughts are true or that they are definitely going to happen.

That's what anxiety does. It completely consumes our thoughts and focus. We become hyperfocused on these thoughts, which prevents us from being able to focus on what is actually happening in the moment. However, those thoughts are oftentimes not valid. We don't always have evidence or proof to show that those thoughts are absolutely, 100 percent true or that negative situations are definitely going to happen. When we become consumed with these thoughts, they take control of our minds. We are so intensely focused on these thoughts that we struggle to focus on what we need to be doing in the moment or identify what is actually within our control. These automatic thoughts make it more difficult to focus on problem-solving or to identify what our priority is in that moment. That's how easily anxiety is triggered and how quickly it can intensify.

We want to pay attention to what we are thinking about in the moments leading up to our anxiety. We want to identify our automatic thoughts that are triggering the anxiety. This takes practice. Because we are not always consciously aware of what we are thinking, we have to try to identify or pay attention to any possible worry or concern that is causing us stress. What are we anticipating? What are we afraid of happening? Identify all those what-if statements. The more we pay attention to our thoughts, the easier it becomes to identify our anxiety-provoking automatic thoughts.

Once we are able to identify these triggering thoughts, we want to ask ourselves, *Do I have any evidence to prove that these thoughts are absolutely true or that something bad is definitely going to happen?* If we don't have proof that our automatic thoughts are absolutely true, we want to then shift our focus to what we are doing in the moment. We need to focus on what our priorities are and manage one thing at a time: *What am I in control of right now? What's the first thing I need to do right now?* This is the cognitive work. We are training our brains to think differently than the way they've been used to thinking throughout our lives. We are reconditioning our brains to think in a more logical, step-by-step manner, and our brains aren't used to doing this on their own. Our brains naturally feed into those anxiety-provoking thoughts that then take over our focus. We are now trying to shift our focus from those anxiety-provoking thoughts to what is actually happening in the moment.

Other examples of assumptions or anticipatory thoughts that we often take on (or internalize, developing core beliefs) and, therefore, trigger our anxiety include but are not limited to the following:

- Fear of being judged, being scrutinized, being embarrassed, being rejected, offending others, etc.
  o If we are fearful of something happening, we are not going to feel we have control in that situation. Fear is an emotional response to a real or perceived threat.
- Anticipation of a future threat.
  o Again, if we feel threatened in any way or anticipate something threatening, we will not feel we have control, or we will feel that the control we have may be taken away.
- Misinterpretation of information.
  o If we misinterpret information, it leads to assuming something that may not necessarily be true.
- Things do not go as planned.
  o If something does not turn out the way we expected, our sense of control drops. We need to be able to accept that plan A did not work out and identify other options that we can use instead or identify another time when we will be able to pursue plan A. If we are able to accept that things do not go as planned and shift our focus to what our other options may be, we are increasing our sense of control in those given circumstances, rather than perseverating on what went wrong and continuing to feel angry or upset by the current circumstances.
- Occurrence of any changes, particularly unexpected changes.
- New experiences.
- Environmental factors (e.g., noises, crowds, or activity).

- Refusal to take accountability for our actions or decisions.
  - o If we justify our behaviors or choices, blame others, manipulate, or make excuses as to why we act inappropriately or make a mistake, we are not taking the correct steps to control the situation.
- Nonacceptance of what is not within our control.
  - o Counterintuitively, if we accept or embrace the fact that some things are out of our control can actually be empowering and freeing, a weight lifted off our shoulders.

Each of these precipitants will be addressed in greater detail later in the book.

Let's look at some other examples of how core beliefs are developed and lay the foundation for our automatic thoughts. Here is an example of a young child, Jane, who accidentally spills her milk at the dinner table. The spill itself can surprise anyone at the table, which can spark a host of reactionary responses. The mother, who happens to be sitting at the table, reacts in a negative way, such as shouting the child's name or exclaiming, "Jane! Come on! Why did you do that?"

Jane may interpret that situation in a way where she assumes she did something bad or wrong and may assume that she disappointed her mother. Jane may also think that what she did was stupid or clumsy; therefore, she is stupid and clumsy. Even though her mom did not state in those words that she is stupid or clumsy, Jane may interpret her mother's reaction as such and is vulnerable to believing this about herself. Jane is likely going to place more value on her mother's immediate reaction rather than recognizing that it was an accident, that she didn't intentionally do anything wrong, and that her mother was just frustrated at the situation and reacted poorly. Children, like adults, are more likely to remember how someone or an event made them feel than what was specifically said to them at the time.

They are also likely to assume that if someone reacts to them in a shocking or aggressive manner, that they must have done something to deserve it. Because they don't have the life skills and experience to know otherwise, they assume that what another person is telling them is true. Young Jane may never express her thoughts—younger kids tend not to speak up about how they are feeling or how they interpret a situation as they may not yet have the tools to do so—but she will likely internalize certain assumptions based on her experience. If she has enough similar experiences, these assumptions can form a core belief about herself that she will carry for the rest of her life.

As a result, Jane, as well as any other child, is very vulnerable to internalizing negative thoughts about themselves. If Jane never speaks up about how she is feeling or what she is thinking, these negative thoughts will not be corrected and will form her core beliefs of who she feels she is and how she identifies herself. Children will start to form a negative sense of self rather than a positive sense of self, which will allow them to feel they are able to exercise a greater sense of control (even though kids are not consciously aware of this development). As children continue to harbor these negative core beliefs throughout their development and into adulthood, any vulnerable situation that taps into their core beliefs will automatically trigger (false) assumptions that they are a disappointment, stupid, not good enough, a failure, etc. These beliefs can stay with them and affect how they see themselves and how they approach challenges throughout their lives.

If I've always believed that I've been a disappointment to others throughout my development, then I'm going to continue to assume this in other aspects of my adult life. I'm going to assume that I'm a disappointment as a spouse, as a parent, as an employee, as a friend, as a daughter, etc., even if evidence suggests otherwise. These negative core beliefs and assumptions will impede my ability to focus on what I am capable of accomplishing, to believe that I'm good enough as I am regardless of accomplishments, or to believe that I actually have the ability to exercise control in my own life.

Another example of how core beliefs form the basis of our anxiety is if a child, Rebecca, gets a grade on a test or in a class that is less than what her parents desire. Rebecca's parents may respond in a way that highlights a lack of accomplishment rather than focusing on what she is actually able to accomplish.

"Why didn't you get an A? Didn't you study enough? What grades did your classmates get?" These questions are examples of the detrimental comments we often make to our kids with regard to their academic performance.

These comments and questions can be interpreted by Rebecca as "I'm not smart enough. I didn't work hard enough. I'm not as smart as my classmates," as well as "My parents are disappointed in me. I'm not good enough for them. They think I'm stupid."

If our kids interpret these experiences in such a negative way, specifically reflecting on how they are stupid or not good enough, or if they feel they failed their parents, they are then vulnerable to internalizing these thoughts, forming core beliefs, and believing these thoughts are true about who they are as a person. They can easily carry these core beliefs with them throughout their lives until they are able to identify them as flawed beliefs or have other corrective experiences that prove these beliefs are not, in fact, true. Let's fast-forward to when Rebecca is an adult. If she grows up internalizing the message that her performance in school is not good enough or that she hasn't accomplished what she should or what's been expected of her, she may become highly focused on accomplishments. She may try to prove her worth by being the best student, super mom, super employee, etc. and not realize that she is good enough and doesn't have to kill herself trying to be perfect, an unattainable goal. If Rebecca is not exceptional at everything she does, she may easily interpret what she does or who she is as a failure.

Triggers

Even though our anxiety is often rooted in core beliefs that are developed when we are young, anxiety can also be triggered by circumstances that may not necessarily be related to our core beliefs or sense of self. An example of how easily anxiety can be triggered and quickly escalate is a student who has a test tomorrow. Jack doesn't feel prepared for his math test. The first automatic thought that pops into his head is *I'm going to fail the test.* That automatic thought can trigger the next thought and so on: *If I fail this test, I'm going to fail the class. If I fail this class, I'm going to fail this semester. If I fail this semester, my GPA is going to drop, and I'm going to have to take summer classes. I'm not going to graduate on time. Colleges aren't going to want to accept me. I'm a failure as a student, which means I'm going to fail in other areas of my life.*

See how easily those thoughts can snowball and escalate the anxiety? Our mind quickly takes us to the worst-case scenario. Jack's anxiety in this example may not necessarily be rooted in his core belief system but is triggered by the circumstances surrounding the issue; Jack is not prepared. However, if Jack develops negative core beliefs when he is younger, based on having experienced negative or critical feedback from his parents or teachers, like the example presented earlier with Rebecca, then Jack's negative core beliefs can trigger anxiety that is not just based on circumstances but is more deeply rooted. Jack may assume he will fail his exam because he is not smart or because he feels he is a failure. He may be more focused on these core beliefs than on recognizing that the anxiety may just be due to the circumstance of not being prepared, therefore, limiting his ability to focus on what is actually within his control or to recognize that these beliefs may not actually be valid. Jack doesn't have proof that he will definitely fail the exam, but he struggles to recognize this or understand how his anxiety is affecting his functioning.

Some automatic thoughts have an obvious source, like not feeling prepared for a test, but others are harder to explain. For example, you may be sitting on the couch after a long, tiring day at school or work. You finally get a chance to relax, but you suddenly start feeling intense anxiety. You may even have a panic attack, but you have no idea why. It feels as though it comes out of nowhere. You are not able to identify any automatic thoughts in the moment because the anxiety is too intense.

Although it may feel as if the anxiety comes out of nowhere, you are feeling this way for a reason. You want to find the source of this anxiety. After the anxiety starts to subside, think back to what you were doing five or ten minutes prior to when the anxiety started. How were you feeling then? Try identifying what you were thinking about at that time. What were you doing? What were you anticipating? Did something you saw, heard, or smelled remind you of a time when you experienced high anxiety?

If you have trouble identifying the triggering automatic thoughts, keep backing yourself up, hour by hour, trying to identify what you were doing and what you were thinking about at the time the anxiety started to set in or what you were doing prior to when you started to feel anxious. Try to recall what you were thinking about. Keep working your way back along the day's timeline until you are able to identify a stressor that potentially triggered the anxiety. Once you work your way back far enough to where you recognize that you were feeling okay and the anxiety wasn't affecting you, think about what might have happened or changed between the time you were feeling okay and when you started to feel anxious. You really want to focus on the automatic thoughts, which can easily be triggered by random experiences throughout your day, including the things you see, hear, smell, or taste; location; environment; people; or responsibilities.

So why do our anxiety or panic symptoms set in out of the blue? Sometimes we may actually have experienced something that can trigger our anxiety earlier in the day, but the anxiety doesn't become overwhelmingly intense right in that moment because we are focusing on our other responsibilities throughout the day. Because we experience so many things throughout our day, much of what we experience is not fully processed by our brain in the moment but is put in the back of our mental filing cabinet. Instead, our brain prioritizes what we are in the middle of doing or what we are anticipating having to do in the immediate future. We don't spend a lot of time processing every single experience or stimulus with which we come in contact throughout the day.

When we sit down at the end of the day to relax and the anxiety sets in, oftentimes, our brain is playing catch-up and processing more information about what we experienced throughout the day. Our brain is now reviewing what we previously put in our mental file cabinet. Our anxiety may not have been triggered in the moment we see someone who looks like someone from our past who will typically spike our anxiety; we are likely more focused on what else has to be done, so we don't think about it too much. But once we sit down to relax at the end of the day, we start to feel panic. It feels like it comes out of nowhere. Our brain is still processing what we see and experience earlier in the day, so our anxiety doesn't intensify until our brain is able to process more information.

I have a client we will refer to as Katie, who is a college student and also works a part-time job. She describes having a panic attack at the end of the day, after getting home from school and work. Katie describes her anxiety as though it were completely random. She isn't doing anything unusual or thinking about anything that makes her particularly anxious and struggles to understand why she will have "random" panic attacks at the end of the day. I have her think back, hour by hour, about what she is doing and how she is feeling. She describes how her day went, including what is being discussed in each of her classes at school. Katie feels her classes went well, and there are good topics and conversations throughout her day.

I ask what topics have been discussed in class. In her criminal justice class, they have watched a video of a man in prison who was in solitary confinement because he was suicidal. When she shares this information with me, she stops talking. She recognizes that the word *suicide* is what triggers her earlier in the day, but the class discussion continues, and she doesn't spend much time focusing on that word in the moment. She then goes throughout the rest of her day, not having processed that her anxiety has been triggered, and because she hasn't focused much on that word or topic in the moment, her brain continues to process that experience well after the fact, which eventually triggers a panic attack.

Once Katie is able to identify the source of her anxiety and the reason for her panic attack, she actually feels a sense of relief. She is able to gain some understanding of her anxiety instead of continuing to feel as if it has come out of nowhere or there is no reason for it.

What Do We Do When We Recognize That Our Automatic Thoughts Are Not Valid?

Once we identify the automatic thoughts that prompt our anxiety, we need to evaluate the validity of these thoughts. Following Judith Beck's recommendations, we will question what evidence we have to support these thoughts. After we identify the automatic thoughts that are triggering our anxiety, we need to ask ourselves, *Do I have any evidence or proof that these thoughts are real? That they are definitely going to happen? Where is the evidence?* When we don't have any proof that these assumptions or anticipatory thoughts are absolutely going to happen, the thoughts are not necessarily valid.

Once we recognize that our thoughts may not be valid, we then want to shift our focus to what we are doing in the moment. Rather than continuing to allow these automatic thoughts to have complete control over our focus, reactions, behaviors, etc., we want to shift our focus from those automatic thoughts to what we are doing in the moment. We need to ask ourselves, *What is my priority right now? What are my responsibilities right now? What is in my best interest right now?* We need to focus on ourselves and what is actually happening in the moment. Our focus needs to be on what is within our control in that moment, not on all the what-ifs that we have no proof will definitely happen.

As we work on shifting our focus from the automatic thoughts to what we are doing in the moment, we are training our brain to think differently than what it's used to. This is the work of the cognitive therapy. We are reconditioning our brain to think in a more logical, step-by-step way, which our brain doesn't typically do on its own. Our brain naturally feeds into the anxiety and allows the anxiety to take complete control of our focus. We become so consumed by our anxiety-provoking thoughts and negative beliefs that we struggle to focus on what we need to be doing in the moment, what our behaviors or actions are, and what is actually within our control.

Shifting our focus from our automatic thoughts to what we are doing in the moment and what we are in control of in the moment takes practice. This is work that we need to do consistently throughout the day to become the masters of our thought processes and not to let them operate on autopilot. We are training our brains to get control of the anxiety-provoking thoughts. We are no longer allowing our anxiety to control our thoughts or what we do. We are taking control of the anxiety by becoming more aware of it, understanding more about what triggers it and where it's rooted, reviewing if our thoughts are valid or not, and shifting our focus to what is within our control.

Judith Beck lists additional questions to evaluate automatic thoughts; however, this is where control theory diverges from cognitive theory. I recommend shifting our focus to what we are doing in the moment after identifying whether these automatic thoughts are valid. I feel it is important to shift our focus to what we can control, given the circumstances. Again, our goal is to recognize what is within our control.

Let's go back to Jack, who is worried about taking a test the next day. If Jack is able to identify and review his automatic thoughts about taking the test and recognizes that he does not have any evidence to prove that his thoughts are valid and that there is no proof to say he is definitely going to fail the exam, we want him to shift his focus back to how he is doing in the present moment. In that moment, he's not failing the exam. In that moment, he's okay. None of his automatic thoughts are happening. He's okay in the moment. Our job is to shift our focus to what our priority is in that moment after identifying our automatic thoughts. However, a more valid thought for the student might be *I'm afraid I won't do well on my exam because I'm not prepared.* This actually leads us to our next step.

What Do We Do When Our Automatic Thoughts Might Be Valid?

If we review our automatic thoughts and find that we are anticipating that something will happen because it's happened before, then those automatic thoughts have some validity. Again, we don't have proof that those anticipatory thoughts are definitely going to happen, but if they do, we want to be able to focus on what we can do to manage the potential situation as best we can. We want to identify options that are within our control to manage the potential situation. In other words, we want to solve the problem.

Maybe Jack, from the last example, is assuming he will fail the test tomorrow because he previously failed a test in that class or with that teacher. In that case, there is some validity to his concern. He may also be anticipating failing the exam because he does not feel prepared. This is also a valid concern. If our automatic thoughts are valid or can potentially happen, then we want to come up with a plan or identify options that are within our control to help manage that potentially stressful situation to the best of our ability. If Jack is worried about failing the test, let's identify some options that are within his control to help prepare as best he can. Keep in mind that even though we are creating a plan to manage the potential situations as best we can, we still don't have proof that he will definitely fail the exam. Some options that are within his control may include the following:

- Carving out time in his schedule that night so he can study
- Reviewing his notes or previous tests from that class
- Reviewing a study guide
- Reviewing the chapters on which he is being tested
- Calling a friend to review some questions
- Making flash cards
- Reviewing vocabulary
- Doing some practice problems

When we are anticipating something that can potentially happen, we want to focus more on problem-solving than continuing to perseverate on our automatic thoughts, which may not ever happen (and are more likely to happen if we are paralyzed with fear).

To do this, we want to start by coming up with plan A that we can implement if a potentially stressful situation presents itself. If plan A doesn't work, go to plan B. If plan B doesn't work, have a plan C.

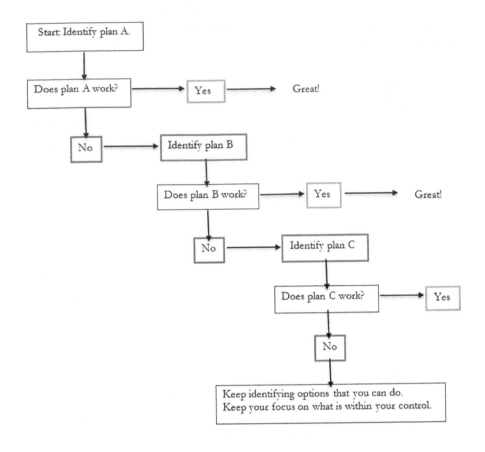

The objective here is to identify options that are within our control and focus on problem-solving. By training ourselves to focus on what is within our control and to identify what our options are to best manage the stressful situation in the moment, we are increasing our sense of control over the situation. As we continue to focus on what our options are, we are training ourselves to engage in more forward thinking and to recognize what is within our control, rather than staying stuck and focusing on what is wrong or not going the way we want.

Also, when we focus on what we can do moving forward, we won't be caught off guard as much as we will be if we don't come up with a plan. We will have already thought through what we can do and will feel more prepared. If we feel more prepared, we will feel a greater sense of control. If we feel a greater sense of control, our anxiety will automatically start to come down on the scale as our confidence and sense of readiness and security increase.

This is also where we exercise flexibility in thinking. We are trying to train ourselves to shift our focus away from what we cannot control toward what we can do in the moment. Judith Beck's cognitive theory puts more focus on the usefulness of automatic thoughts than control theory, in which we aim to focus more on what we can do in the situation, using practical skills and giving ourselves a greater sense of control.

Just because something does not work out the way we want or intend does not mean that we are failures or can't be successful. We have to learn how to accept what doesn't go our way while still holding ourselves accountable for focusing on what else we can do moving forward. One way to help accept what we don't have control over is to ask ourselves, *What is my responsibility right now?* If we can't change the circumstances we are facing, we want to then shift our focus to what we are capable of doing in the moment. What is plan B?

Let's revisit the example where Jack is assuming he is going to fail his exam. In addition to focusing on what his options are to help prepare as best he can, given the time constraint, he may also try accepting that potentially getting a C on the exam is an acceptable goal because getting an A may be unlikely if he doesn't have a lot of time to prepare. We want to practice being flexible in our expectations, given circumstances that are not within our control.

Anticipating the Next Panic Attack or Anxiety Episode

It is very common for people who have had severe anxiety or panic attacks to constantly be anticipating when the next one will happen. This anticipation is another example of how easily we can get caught up in our thoughts and assumptions about something that may not ever come to fruition. However, because of our history with anxiety and panic attacks, the anticipation of another attack has some validity. When we assume that we are going to have another anxiety or panic attack, that thought takes control, and it is very difficult for us to focus on what we are doing in the moment. We struggle to recognize in the moment that we are okay. We need to focus on the fact that we aren't currently having a panic attack and are safe, healthy, etc.

Unfortunately, we continuously anticipate: *What if this happens? What if that happens?* Those thoughts trigger more automatic thoughts about what else may happen if we have a panic attack, and soon, we are focusing on the worst-case scenario. Those thoughts have taken control of us once again, and we struggle to focus on how we are doing or what we need to do in that moment, to be mindful or present.

When we focus so much of our attention on the what-ifs, we struggle to focus on what we are actually doing in the moment. We may be doing something absolutely benign, but we allow ourselves to get caught up in the automatic thoughts that trigger anxiety. Here is where we want to recognize that we are having automatic thoughts. We need to identify those thoughts and review them to see if they are valid. We need to ask ourselves if we have any evidence to prove that these thoughts are absolutely true or that these fears are definitely going to happen. Do we know for a fact that we are definitely going to have another panic attack in the near future? If there is no evidence to support the automatic thoughts, we want to shift our focus from those thoughts to what we are doing in the present moment. We want to focus on what is within our control and what our priority is in that moment, rather than focusing on the what-ifs that may not ever happen.

However, when we are anticipating an anxiety or panic attack, we often assume that because we previously had a panic attack, we're going to have one again. When we base our assumptions on past experiences, it's hard to convince ourselves that it's not going to happen again. Our past experience provides evidence that the experience can, in fact, happen again. In this case, we want to identify what we can do if that situation recurs (if we do have another panic attack) to help us best manage that potential event. Now, we still don't have proof that we are definitely going to have another panic attack in the near future. However, by identifying options that we can utilize should an attack arise, we are increasing our sense of control over the situation. We are getting the automatic thoughts back under control and bringing our anxiety down by creating a plan of action.

For example, if I'm anticipating having a panic attack when I'm in a public setting, I want to identify options to help manage it. Where can I go if I start to feel anxious? Can I step outside and get some space away from the crowded room? Is there someone I feel comfortable talking to if I need to? Maybe I can leave an event early if I become too overwhelmed. I can even lock myself in a bathroom if I need a couple of minutes away from others. These are all options that are within my control.

Keep in mind that we don't want to avoid engaging in social or other events that may trigger anxiety (assuming we aren't engaging in anything too dangerous). Even if we leave an event early, at least we are able to make it to the event. Once there, we should continue to gauge how we're doing from time to time, focusing on how we're able to maintain control. (I will address avoidance in detail when discussing defense mechanisms.) Once we are able to identify options or come up with a plan to help manage that potential situation, we then put that plan aside and shift our focus back to what we are doing in the moment. We need to keep training ourselves to stay focused on how we are feeling in the moment, what we are doing in the moment, what is currently within our control, and what our primary responsibility is at that time. We need to recognize that, in that moment, we aren't having a panic attack, and we are actually still in control.

It can be difficult, particularly at the beginning, to shift our focus from the automatic thoughts to what we are doing in the moment or what our priority is right then. Again, our brains naturally feed into our anxiety-provoking thoughts because it is a natural defense mechanism, better suited to escaping predators than dealing with work deadlines. It's the fight-or-flight reactive response when we feel threatened or feel we do not have sufficient control.

Unfortunately, we can quickly and easily become completely consumed by these automatic thoughts, to the point where it is very difficult to stop focusing on them. In order for us to shift our focus from the automatic thoughts that consume us to what we are doing in the moment, we need to continuously practice this skill until it becomes natural. The cognitive exercises that we will be building on train our brains to think in a more logical, step-by-step manner. The cognitive approach conditions our brains to think differently than they are used to with regard to anxiety. Our brains naturally react to their environment in a defensive manner and feed into our anxiety. This cognitive approach gets easier the more you become familiar with and practice it, but it can take some time to adjust your approach.

PART 3

How Is Control Theory Applied?

Sense of Self and Self-Esteem

Self-esteem is one aspect that is directly affected by anxiety. To better understand this, let's go back to the scale. When our anxiety is high on the scale, our sense of control is low. Self-esteem goes hand in hand with our sense of control. Think about your own confidence when your anxiety is high. If you don't feel you have the level of control you need in a particular situation, your confidence and self-esteem are likely to also be low.

When our anxiety is high, we are vulnerable to negative beliefs, such as the following: *I'm not good enough. I'm not smart enough or as good as others. I'm a disappointment. I'm a failure.* We are vulnerable to internalizing these thoughts if we don't feel we have the level of control that we need or want. If we feel we know what we're doing and have evidence to prove that we're capable of doing or accomplishing something, then our sense of control is going to be higher with regard to that aspect of our lives. Our anxiety will, therefore, be lower; and our self-esteem and confidence will be higher with our increased sense of control. We're not going to be as vulnerable to having these negative thoughts and beliefs if we know what we are capable of and have a higher level of control in a certain area of our lives. Self-esteem isn't just about feeling that we are awesome; it also encompasses understanding ourselves to a greater degree and knowing who we are and what is personally important to us versus who we think others want us to be.

Our sense of self and self-esteem can be analyzed by identifying recurrent themes within our automatic thoughts. These themes will likely stem from the core beliefs that often build the foundation for our anxiety-provoking thoughts. Aaron Beck talks about the ways in which we distort information, creating what we have been referring to as automatic thoughts. The way in which we interpret information can be influenced by our core beliefs. Aaron Beck refers to these themes as "cognitive distortions." He lists several of these—all-or-nothing thinking, catastrophizing, emotional reasoning, etc.—which Judith Beck also includes in her work. Although these thought distortions can differ, there is a common theme among them, which is a lack of sense of control. There is a theme of lacking self-confidence or a positive sense of self within these cognitive distortions; they are based on assumptions or anticipatory thoughts, and they lend a feeling of helplessness or hopelessness, which, again, is lacking a sense of control.

After identifying and evaluating automatic thoughts, Judith Beck focuses on formulating new beliefs. According to Judith Beck, many of our core beliefs are not necessarily truths but are ideas that can be changed or modified. I find this theory helpful and relevant to our own work with automatic thoughts, specifically for those who often present with rigid, all-or-nothing thinking. Some of these beliefs or ideas that Judith Beck presents in her work have been very common in my work with clients:

- If I don't do as well as others, I'm a failure.
- If I ask for help, it's a sign of weakness.
- If I fail at work or school, I'm a failure as a person.
- I should be able to excel at everything I try.
- If I don't live up to my potential, I have failed.
- If I don't work hard all the time, I'll fail.
- If I show my emotions or cry, I'm weak.

At the root of these thoughts are core beliefs, which also lay the groundwork for our self-worth. If we have negative experiences as a child, which we interpret as letting down someone important in our lives (such as feeling like we have disappointed our parents), we may have misinterpreted that experience and, therefore, become vulnerable to believing that we are not good enough or that we don't live up to our parents' expectations in a more universal sense. If we don't talk to our parents about these thoughts and feelings (as children very rarely do) and don't receive any feedback to help correct our interpretation of that experience, help us understand that we did not fail but that maybe we made the wrong choice, and help us learn from the situation, we will likely carry this core belief with us into other areas of our lives and throughout our development.

If we grow up believing that we're never going to meet anyone's expectations or that we're going to fail at most things we pursue, we will continue to experience high levels of anxiety and automatically take on negative assumptions in different areas of our lives. We will have a difficult time feeling confident that we will be able to succeed, or at least not fail or suffer a humiliating outcome, in whatever we try. We will also have a harder time accepting that, even if we don't perform up to the level we were expecting, it does not mean that we're failures or that we won't be able to accomplish our goals.

Furthermore, we need to think about what our goals and values are. Our primary goal should always be to do our best. If we know that we are doing our best, then we are doing our job. Simultaneously, we want to be flexible with ourselves if we don't perform better than others around us. We are not failures if others have outperformed us when we know we have done the best we can. We can still hold ourselves accountable and continue working hard to improve our skills. We need to become aware of our automatic thoughts, as well as to explore the underlying core beliefs that lay the foundation for these thoughts. When we increase our level of awareness of our thought processes and beliefs, we are better equipped to evaluate the validity of these thoughts and prevent ourselves from internalizing negative, self-deprecating thoughts.

Let's review where our anxiety is when we are flooded with automatic thoughts. When our minds become consumed by automatic thoughts, our anxiety quickly becomes higher on the scale. When our anxiety is high on the scale, our sense of control has dropped. Again, if we feel we have more control over a given situation, we won't be as vulnerable to assuming or anticipating something that may not ever come to fruition, and therefore, our anxiety will not be as high on the scale.

So where is our self-esteem when all this is going on? When we don't have a healthy, strong sense of control over a situation or over one or more aspects of our lives, our self-esteem also drops. When our anxiety is high on the scale and our sense of control is low, our self-esteem is right down there with our sense of control. They go hand in hand. As we start to exercise more control over a situation or one or more aspects of our lives, our self-esteem is going to increase. As we see more evidence that we are effectively communicating or setting boundaries with others, and as others are starting to respond to us more appropriately, we're going to feel our sense of control increase, as well as our confidence, as we're seeing for ourselves that we're doing the work and creating the positive changes we desire. We're going to feel more confident in ourselves that when another stressful situation arises, we will know what we're capable of doing or what we need to do. We will feel more prepared and more confident and have an increased sense of control.

An example of how our self-esteem suffers as a result of our anxiety is when we are dealing with social interactions. It is very common for people to experience heightened anxiety in social situations. When we are interacting with others—more specifically, people with whom we are not necessarily well acquainted—we tend to presume how others are perceiving us. We often start focusing automatically on what others think of us, leading to automatic thoughts, such as the following: *Do they like me? Am I making a good impression? Do they think I'm smart? Do they think I'm interesting? Do they like how I look? They think I'm stupid. I'm so annoying. They don't want to talk to me. They're not going to want to hang out with me again.* The thoughts go on and on.

If we're already assuming that these thoughts are true, our sense of control is quickly lowered, if it isn't already low before, and our self-esteem is also low. We aren't going to feel confident in ourselves or be fully engaged in the social situation if we are so focused on these negative automatic thoughts, potentially leading to the negative impression we are worried about making.

56

Body image is another area that is affected by the way in which we perceive or interpret information and feedback from others, affecting our self-esteem. A lot of people, especially adolescents, are highly focused on what others think of them and try to look a certain way in order to be accepted, approved, or not judged negatively. We also see so much in the media and society in general that emphasizes the need or expectation for everyone to look thin and stylish. When it's constantly in our faces, it's hard to ignore.

Unfortunately, our anxiety can easily feed into the need to meet others' expectations, including those of people we don't even know. Again, this is why it is so critical for us to focus on ourselves and what is in our own best interest. When we place so much focus on others' expectations and allow others to influence what we do, what we wear, what we eat, or how much we weigh in ways that are not healthy or appropriate, we are allowing others to have a level of control over us that is not serving our best interests. In those moments, when we make a choice to dress a certain way or control what we eat so that we can fit in with others or be accepted, we are exercising a false sense of control. Our anxiety may decrease slightly on the scale, but it's only temporary, and we're not exercising healthy control of ourselves. We need to focus on what is right for ourselves and what makes us feel comfortable and authentic, not what we think others expect of us or what society tells us we should look like.

We are in control of our own bodies, no one else. It is not up to anyone else what we do, what we eat, what we wear, how much we weigh, or how we present our sexuality or gender identity. We need to focus on how we exercise control over our own bodies and how we take care of ourselves. If we don't fit a certain societal mold but we know that we're taking care of ourselves in the way we need to and stay focused on making most decisions in our best interests, then we are doing our job. It's not up to anyone else to control how we choose or how we take care of ourselves. If we are too focused on how others are judging us with regard to our physical appearance, our sense of control drops, and our self-esteem also takes a hit. If we're allowing others to influence how we look in order to feel approved or accepted—in other words, to control us—then we're not exactly feeling confident in ourselves, thus limiting our self-esteem.

Additionally, if others care so much and feel the need to judge us, it actually speaks more to their own anxieties, insecurities, and limited self-esteem and is not our anxiety to hold. Here is where we need to be mindful of when it may not necessarily be our anxiety but someone else's. In that case, we are not responsible for managing others' anxieties. We are responsible for taking care of ourselves and our own health, not someone else's anxiety.

For those who have battled disordered eating and are in recovery, think about how your way of thinking has changed since you last engaged in disordered eating. What are you focused on with regard to your own body and health? It's common for those who are in recovery to learn to appreciate their bodies as they are: that they don't have to look a certain way or the way in which society tells you. Think about what is happening in this change of thought. You are shifting your focus from them to you. You are taking back your personal sense of control that is once lost to others, trying to look the way you think others want you to or weigh what you think is acceptable to others.

When we are so focused on what we think others want us to look like, wear, or weigh, we are essentially giving them our personal sense of control. When we shift our focus back to ourselves, we are taking back that control. We are deciding that we have control over our bodies, not anyone else. We are not allowing others to control what we look like. We learn to love ourselves for who we are and recognize that we are not going to let others make decisions for us regarding how we look or feel about ourselves. We stop allowing others to have that control over us, and we learn to exercise healthy control for ourselves. We learn to stay focused on ourselves and appreciate ourselves. When we are too focused on what others think of us, we often lose sight of what makes us unique. We let others destroy what makes us special. However, when we shift our focus back to ourselves, we stop allowing others to take away or minimize what makes us unique. We learn to appreciate who we are individually, and we will not let others define who we are or who we should be.

WHY ON EARTH DO I FEEL THIS WAY?

(Eating disorders are also a type of defense mechanism, which I will address further in the reading.)

Lastly, if others can't accept that we look different from them (including in ways that are not within our control, such as skin color or other physical attributes), then they are responsible for accepting that they can't control others and that not everyone is going to agree with them. Here is where we need to set a mental boundary for ourselves, recognizing that others have to learn to accept what is not within their control and to focus on themselves as well. It is not our job to look or present ourselves in a certain way to fit another's expectations. Even if others are not able to accept what is not within their control or focus on themselves, it's still important that we at least set a mental boundary for ourselves, knowing that we are not doing anything wrong if we don't meet someone else's expectations. Again, if we are taking care of ourselves in the ways that are in our best interests, then we are doing our job. We are the only ones who control how we take care of our bodies and how we present ourselves, no one else.

Meeting Expectations

Expectations, those of others as well as our own, can be very stressful and anxiety provoking. Young kids frequently try to please their parents, caregivers, teachers, and other important adult figures in their lives. Expectations can also stem from our core beliefs. By becoming more aware of our core beliefs, we are better equipped to catch our automatic thoughts and less likely to misinterpret feedback based on our core beliefs (not assume the worst or that someone is only giving us negative feedback). Our focus on body image may not even start in adolescence. If we are exposed to information relating to body image or hear comments about how we look when we are young, we can easily misinterpret that information and start to internalize negative (automatic) thoughts about ourselves.

If a child hears someone who is important to them making comments about how they or someone else looks, or even makes a comment to the child about their appearance, the child can easily interpret these comments in a way that is damaging to their own sense of self. The child may start to wonder if that person they idolize disapproves of how they look. These early experiences, depending on how a child interprets them, can start to mold their core beliefs that others won't approve of them. These core beliefs will continue throughout their development until the child, adolescent, or even adult becomes aware of how their beliefs have affected their sense of self and recognizes how these core beliefs have been triggering negative automatic thoughts in any circumstance where they feel vulnerable about their appearance. Until we gain awareness of these core beliefs and their impact on our anxiety, our sense of control remains limited.

When we focus on ourselves, we are working on building our sense of self-worth. We learn about our own strengths and weaknesses and what we are capable of accomplishing. When we are more focused on ourselves, we are better equipped not to let others' judgments interfere with or exercise control over what we need to do for ourselves. We also learn not to compare ourselves to others. Comparing ourselves to others shifts our sense of control from ourselves to them, making us vulnerable to putting unrealistic expectations on ourselves. When we do not meet these expectations, we often interpret this as a failure. Focusing on our needs is not the same as being self-centered. It can help us appreciate that the way in which others act, dress, etc. is their way of meeting their own needs. We can then accept each other as unique individuals.

Another example of how we often allow others to have control over us is when we anticipate how others may react to something we say or do. Oftentimes, we will avoid doing or saying something because we are afraid of upsetting another person. Our intention is not to upset anyone, but it is important that we can express what we need to say. However, when we avoid doing or saying something because we are anticipating how another person will react, we are giving them our control.

Referring back to the scale, our anxiety increases when we anticipate how that person is going to react, so if we avoid that conversation or behavior, our anxiety will temporarily go down on the scale, once again giving us a false sense of control. Unfortunately, our actual level of control stays low because we are still allowing that other person to hold the control and influence what we do. Eventually, that anxiety is going to go back up on the scale because we don't actually manage the situation and exercise control in an effective manner. We aren't focusing on ourselves but on others' potential reactions (although we have no definitive evidence of how they will react), and therefore, we are letting go of our own sense of control. (I will address avoidance at greater length when discussing defense mechanisms.)

One critical example of how expectations can spike anxiety is when adolescents are undergoing the college application process. Ask any student nowadays what their experience has been when thinking about what colleges to which they will or have applied. This process has changed significantly since the 1990s and early 2000s. Students are under extreme stress when going through this process: starting with just thinking about the schools they will apply to, their SAT or ACT scores, their GPA, the level classes they take, and the many extracurricular activities they are involved in; being captain or top athlete on their sports team; getting scouted by different schools; applying for scholarships; and the list goes on. (Not to mention the pressure that parents often place on their kids to get into a top school.)

This is just the tip of the iceberg when students are preparing for college. The underlying automatic thoughts on which the students perseverate are guiding them to make decisions that may not necessarily be in their best interests or even make them happy. Students are taking on expectations from others all around them. They are more focused on what others want them to do than on what they feel is right for them. They want to make their parents proud and get accepted into top-tier schools. They constantly compare themselves to their peers, which leads them to feel or assume that they are not as smart as their peers, based on their grades or test scores. They assume they won't get into as good a school as their friends, which further leads them to assume that they won't be as successful as their peers, they won't get a good job, they won't be able to buy a home, etc. and that others will perceive them as failures. When students are constantly comparing themselves to their peers or focusing on what they think their parents, teachers, or others want them to do, they are essentially giving others control over their decision-making processes and their lives. They are only focusing on what they think others want or expect them to do, rather than focusing on themselves and what is actually in their best interests.

It's also common for students to view this process in all-or-nothing terms: *If I don't get into the school of my choice, then what's the point of pursuing any school. I'm just a failure.* Students have a very difficult time recognizing that if they don't get into the school of their choice, they can still choose another school and be just as successful and happy, perhaps even more so. But because a student doesn't get into their first-choice school, they automatically assume that they won't be as successful in life and that others will be better off.

We need to communicate with our kids and students that they are the ones in control of where they apply and what they pursue. They are becoming adults and need to exercise their own independent choices. Parents need to let their kids exercise this control. If students choose not to hold themselves accountable for their responsibilities (for example, they don't get their applications in on time), then they need to learn from the natural consequences. Parents cannot be doing the work for their kids, and by "work," I mean organizing their college information, filling out college applications, signing them up for SATs or ACTs, getting transcripts or letters of recommendations for their kids, doing homework for them, etc. Students need to focus on what is important to them personally and not what is important to others—peers or adults. If they are hardworking students and are able to hold themselves accountable for their responsibilities, then they are doing their job. Those skills and the ability to focus on themselves will transfer to other aspects of their lives, whether they attend college, go into the workforce, raise a family, etc. If students don't get accepted into the schools of their choice, it does not mean that they will not be successful in life. It does not mean that they will never get accepted into college. It does not mean they are failures. There is no evidence to prove that these will be the outcomes. They will be okay if they don't get accepted into their first-choice school. They are also capable of coming up with alternate plans if plan A or plan B doesn't work out.

Furthermore, students often allow colleges to exercise control over what they should be doing. For example, students take on the expectations of schools where they have to get a certain score on their SAT or ACT to be considered or they need to have a GPA of 3.8 or higher, and even students who have a 4.0 GPA are getting rejected from schools. This is absurd. A GPA does not define how successful a student is or will be later in life. However, students take these expectations to heart and feel that, if they don't have the GPA or test score a school is expecting, they are not good enough or, once again, a failure. Students are allowing colleges to have control over what they do with their lives, rather than focusing on what is in their best interests.

Students need to be focusing on themselves and asking themselves, *What is going to make me happy? Where do I want to go? What am I interested in pursuing in school or as a career? What am I passionate about? What do I want to explore?* It's not up to the college to determine if you are good enough. I always encourage my clients to focus on how they can exercise control when interviewing with colleges or even jobs. Students need to ask schools (or at least think about), "What do you have to offer me? Convince me that I want to come to your school. What am I going to walk away with after my time at your school? How is this school or job going to help enhance my career and what I want to pursue?" Students need to shift the power of control from the schools to themselves. They are in control of their future, not the schools or anyone else. Regardless of what others want or expect from our students, they need to learn how to navigate the world based on their own choices and to focus on what is important to them, not on what they think others want from them.

Social Media

Another prime example of how easy it is for us to lose focus on ourselves, triggering severe anxiety and affecting our self-esteem, is social media. We are exposed to what others are doing, good and bad, and we make judgments about others, or we assume others are judging us. We are able to present to others what we want them to see and, therefore, allow others to control what we do or how we present ourselves. People frequently present their best moments on social media, and we then assume all their moments are amazing. We judge our blah moments against their top 1 percent moments. We are more focused on what others think of us than on ourselves. As we become more consumed with what others think of us, we are less able to develop our own personal sense of who we are. We base our sense of self on how we think others judge us or on assumptions we have of how others perceive us. Once again, we are letting others control who we think we should be and are not focused on ourselves or what is important to us.

A study found that when children, teens, and young adults consistently spend excessive time on social media, they feel increasingly lonely, tired, and left out (Twenge 2017). A study conducted by Dr. Jean Twenge, author of *iGen*, focused on the impact of smartphones on adolescents between 2011 and 2012, when the number of those owning smartphones increased to more than 50 percent. She had started doing research on generational differences twenty-five years before. The study found the following:

- There was a significant increase in the number of kids who said they felt sad, hopeless, and useless and felt that they couldn't do anything right, etc.
- There was an increased number of kids felt left out and lonely.
- There was a 50 percent increase in the number of cases of clinically diagnosed depression between 2011 and 2015.
- There was a significant increase in the suicide rate compared to prior years.
- There was nearly 40 percent of eighth, tenth, and twelfth graders who got less than seven hours of sleep.
- There was a significant decrease in the number of eighth, tenth, and twelfth graders spending time with their friends in person.

These findings are not surprising when applying control theory in how we perceive information. We automatically start making assumptions that are not necessarily true. We are more intensely focused on what others are doing or how we think others are perceiving us than we are on ourselves. When we see what others are doing on social media, we assume we are intentionally left out or that our friends do not want to include us. This is what adolescents refer to as FOMO or "fear of missing out." We become consumed by what others think rather than focus on ourselves and what makes us happy. We end up acting in ways that are not true to ourselves. Our actions are based on what we think others want us to do, or we act in ways to please others rather than focusing on what's in our own best interest. When we aren't focused on ourselves, we don't feel we have the level of control we need; therefore, our anxiety automatically increases.

Older generations didn't typically know (at least not immediately) if there was a get-together that they weren't invited to. They didn't see pictures of each time people went out or engaged in social activities. They didn't put as much focus on what they looked like when they were hanging out with their friends because they were the only ones there, and they didn't have cameras in their pockets.

Consider bullying. We didn't used to have to worry about being bullied once we left school. Home was a safe place where we weren't bullied by our peers. Even if we were bullied, not everyone saw it. It wasn't exposed to everyone to humiliate us in the public eye. Now, everyone can see who's being bullied, and they often just follow what's happening or join in the bullying. It's a completely different world compared to even twenty years ago.

Cyberbullying has also been a significant catalyst for controlling and manipulating others. There have been several incidents in which cyberbullying has been a contributing factor in people committing suicide. Oftentimes, cyberbullies are exposing others' private lives and stripping people of their own personal sense of control. They use this personal information to blackmail or manipulate people to get what they want or simply to make others feel so vulnerable that it becomes excruciatingly painful and overwhelming, and they don't know what to do, leading them to take their own lives so they don't have to live under the extreme control of someone else.

Where does our control go in these instances of social anxiety? We are not focusing on ourselves. We are focused on what other people think of us and are allowing others to hold that control over us. We need to recognize our automatic thoughts when we find ourselves in stressful social circumstances and review these thoughts: Do we have any evidence or proof that these assumptions are absolutely true? Do we know for a fact that others definitely feel one way or another about us? We can't predict what others are thinking, and more often than not, we don't have evidence to prove that others are definitely judging us in a negative way. Unfortunately, we become so consumed by these thoughts that we start to believe they are true before exploring any evidence to support them. Again, when our sense of control is low, our self-esteem also suffers.

Now let's use an example of a social scenario where we feel a stronger sense of control. Let's say we are going to a party for a friend. (This can be relevant for any age.) We may have an idea about who may be there because we know who our friend enjoys seeing socially. Not to mention that we will know the person we will be celebrating. There may be a little anxiety because we may not know everyone there, but we have an idea of who may be there that we know. We may even reach out to some of these friends before the party to see if they are going, giving us a better sense of who will be there. When we have more information about the situation we will be going into, we will likely feel more control than we would if we don't know who is going to be there or whether we will know anyone.

Just having a little more information about what (or who) to expect will give us a stronger sense of control. We will automatically have more of a plan of what we can do and who we can talk to at the party. If we know who we will be able to talk to at the party, we will be less likely to focus on how others may be judging us or to assume others are thinking negatively about us, and our anxiety will likely not be extremely high on the scale. We will also be less likely to distort or misinterpret social interactions if we know more about the people with whom we are engaging.

We will be less likely to allow the influence of others to affect our own sense of self or our behaviors. We will feel more confident saying no to doing something we don't want to do, such as drinking or using drugs. When we know what to expect, our anxiety will be lower; therefore, we will have a better sense of control and be likely to feel more confident in ourselves. This makes sense when you think about meeting new people. Initially, we may feel a bit anxious when speaking with someone for the first time, but once we get to know that person better, we feel more relaxed because we know more about them and how we can relate to or engage with them. We gain a better sense of control.

Flexibility in Thinking

Because we are so vulnerable to misinterpreting or distorting information, we want to pay attention to these thoughts when we set out to attain a goal but are not able to meet our own (and oftentimes others') expectations. Just like with automatic thoughts, we want to evaluate these cognitive distortions to see if there is any evidence that these beliefs are valid or not. Our all-or-nothing thinking, black-and-white thinking, catastrophizing, generalizing, etc. may not necessarily be valid. Once we are able to identify these thoughts or beliefs, we then want to identify alternative outcomes or explanations that can potentially happen.

Here is another example of where we are practicing flexibility in thinking. Flexibility in thinking is being able to modify our plans or options as needed. We are training our brains to think in the gray area. By exercising more flexibility in our thinking, we are able to focus on the pertinent information at hand, rather than on the potential negative feedback, allowing us to stay focused on ourselves, our accomplishments, and the things we are able to do moving forward, and focus on what is within our control and what we are able to problem solve.

Just because we don't get an A on a test does not automatically mean that we have failed or that we're not smart. We may have made a mistake and don't catch it. We may have read the question wrong. Maybe we think we are more prepared than we actually are. Maybe we are exhausted when we take the test and aren't able to focus.

In any case, we want to focus on what we learn from the experience. If we don't get as high a grade as we will have liked or are expecting, we want not just to understand the possible reasons we don't perform well, but also to identify what we can do differently next time. We want to focus on what we can do moving forward, rather than perseverating on the thought or belief that we failed. We also want to recognize that it is okay not to always get As on our exams. We can still make that a goal, but we need to allow ourselves to be more reasonable and flexible with our expectations of ourselves. If we don't get an A on a test, it does not mean that we're not smart or that we're a failure. We can still pass the class. The test or grade does not define who we are or what we are capable of accomplishing. We want to focus on the fact that we did what we could or the best we could in the situation. Granted, there may be times when we didn't put all our effort into doing the best we could and maybe slacked off; in which case, we need to take accountability for these choices. (I will address accountability in greater detail later in the reading.)

An example of utilizing flexibility in thinking and a solution-focused approach is going about a typical day of work. We leave the house at the usual time, but while we are en route, there is an unexpected traffic standstill on a main road of our commute. Initially, we may feel frustrated as our usual routine is not going as planned. Here is where we have to accept that we don't have control over the traffic or what is happening on the road and shift our focus to what our other options are. What are some of the concerns (automatic thoughts) that pop into our heads when we first approach the standstill? We may first be wondering what is causing the standstill (and hoping that no one is hurt if there is an accident), but we may also be assuming that we will be late for work, and this can possibly ruin our morning.

Now we don't have proof that we will definitely be late for work, so let's shift our focus and identify the options that are within our control, given the circumstances. We can come up with another plan to get to work. By coming up with an alternate plan, our sense of control will increase, and our anxiety will automatically start to decrease. When we are able to be flexible in our thinking, we aren't so rigid and stuck on the fact that there is a traffic jam, and we don't continue to sit in the traffic feeling angry. If we are familiar with the area, we may know some back roads we can take to work. We can also ask for directions or use GPS. We can also call our employer to inform them that we may be late due to a traffic incident, so we don't worry about what our supervisor is going to say if we are actually late. This also prevents our supervisor from making assumptions about why we are late or thinking that we are being irresponsible. These are all options that are within our control when things do not go according to our initial plan.

Another example of focusing on what is within our control and using flexibility in thinking is when we want to exercise, but we have no energy or motivation. We may feel that if we don't put in a full-hour workout, there is no point in exercising at all. It's all or nothing. Here, as well, we need to modify our expectations. Instead of focusing on the all-or-nothing thinking, let's come up with a more manageable plan. If we don't feel like going to the gym today, maybe we can just work out for ten or fifteen minutes, then assess how we feel. If we're still too tired and don't have energy, we still got in ten or fifteen minutes of a workout instead of not going at all. If we feel good after ten or fifteen minutes, then we can try to do ten or fifteen minutes more, then see how we feel again. Instead of giving up from the start and not even attempting to exercise, we may actually prove that we're able to accomplish a lot more than we think we can, just by challenging ourselves with manageable small steps.

We can also apply this approach to studying or working. When we are presented with a big task or project, it may feel overwhelming. We may automatically question if we are capable of successfully completing this work. Even though the project may seem challenging, we don't want to assume that we won't be able to complete the project or do a good job. We don't have any proof of not being able to do the work. We may be challenged by our core beliefs or previous experiences when we may not have performed up to our or someone else's expectations and, therefore, interpret that experience as a failure or assume that others do not feel we are suitable or smart enough for the job. We need to pay attention to these thoughts and ask ourselves if we have any evidence or proof that we definitely won't succeed with this project. Even though we may not have proof that we won't be successful, we still may feel overwhelmed. So how do we manage to take on such a big task? Break it down:

- We can use a planner to schedule time each day that we can dedicate to working on the project. Laying out a schedule can help prevent procrastination. Within this schedule, we may even break our work down into smaller tasks. We may start with doing research one week, then coming up with an outline of how to present this information, then writing the paper or constructing the project, then using the remaining blocks of time to review the work and make any needed changes.

- Even during times of studying or working, we may have a hard time focusing. In that case, we can start out by doing twenty to thirty minutes of work, then take a break. Then go back and do twenty to thirty more minutes of work and take another break. Our natural attention span is actually quite limited. We are better able to refocus after taking a break and then coming back to the task at hand than if we try to force ourselves to focus for long periods of time. The way our memory works is that we are likely to remember more information at the start of a studying or reading period and the end. If we break our studying or reading periods into shorter segments, we are increasing the amount of information we are likely to retain.

  However, if we sit down to study for an hour or two hours straight, we will most likely remember more information at the start of that hour and the end, but there is a lot more time in the middle where we are less likely to retain as much information. When we break these study periods into smaller segments, we will still remember more information at the start and the end of those segments, but we are limiting the amount of information in the middle of that study period that we won't remember.

By identifying a plan, organizing our tasks, and managing our time, we have more control over managing the project. These are important objectives in managing larger tasks that initially feel overwhelming. When we utilize our organizational and time-management skills, our sense of control increases, which automatically decreases our anxiety and overwhelming feelings. As our sense of control increases, our confidence also increases. Our self-esteem and confidence are directly related to our sense of control. When we see ourselves accomplishing these tasks that we planned out and organized, we have evidence in front of us that proves we are capable of successfully completing our work.

It is also important for us to focus on areas of success, accomplishments, and progress. We want to shift our focus from the negative core beliefs to any area where there is concrete evidence of progress or success. Unfortunately, it is very easy to let the anxiety take control and focus more on our negative aspects and qualities than to pay attention to anything positive we may have accomplished. Following are examples:

- I really didn't feel like going to the gym today, but I was able to go for an abbreviated workout.
- I didn't clean the windows in the house today, but I was able to clean all the bathrooms, do the laundry, vacuum, and clean the floors.
- I didn't get as much work done today as I wanted to, but I was at least able to organize myself so I am prepared for tomorrow and the rest of this week.

If we have a better sense of control going into the next day or the upcoming week, we will feel more confident in our own ability to succeed in our work. Unfortunately, it is very easy to lose sight of all the things we have accomplished or areas of progress. We tend to focus on the one thing that we didn't do or failed to get done.

These examples show how easy it is for us to interpret information in a way that impedes our ability to focus on what we are able to accomplish, recognize what is within our control, or understand

73

that we did the best we could. It also points out how damaging it can be to our sense of self and self-confidence when the focus of the situation is on what we did not do, rather than what we were able to accomplish. When we repeatedly hear comments that focus on how we are not meeting others' expectations, we are likely to develop a thought pattern that becomes focused on what other people expect of us, which are as follows:

1. Prevents us from being able to focus on ourselves
2. Makes us constantly change or modify our behaviors and what we say, based on what we think other people want us to do or what we think they want to hear
3. Allows others to ultimately control what we do

We are not focusing on what is in our own control or what we feel we need to do that is in our own best interests.

An exercise that I often recommend to my clients is to do a nightly self-check-in before going to bed, identifying all the areas of progress, success, and accomplishment they achieved throughout the day. These areas of success can be something small, such as the following:

- finally having the time to run to the post office
- scheduling an oil change for your car
- finishing a book
- making it to the gym
- making dinner
- taking a shower (parents especially know what I mean)

It can also be something big, such as the following:

- completing a large part of a project you've been working on for school or work
- doing a presentation
- taking care of your kids all day
- managing a classroom of kids

- running a race
- getting a promotion

We need to practice focusing on what we are capable of accomplishing and validating our strengths and accomplishments. It is important that we do not minimize the work that we do and how we have succeeded.

Focusing on Ourselves

The examples we've been discussing highlight one of the most critical tools for managing anxiety and increasing our personal sense of control, which is to focus on ourselves. This objective takes practice. It is so easy for us to focus on what others expect of us, making other people happy, not making anyone upset or disappointing others that we forget to focus on ourselves. Remember, it is important to recognize that when we focus so much on what others want and not what we want, we end up acting in ways or making decisions that aren't necessarily in our best interests. By doing so, we are giving others our control. If we allow others to exercise this control over us (even though it's not necessarily intentional on their part), we won't feel comfortable or authentic because we aren't acting on our own behalf. Therefore, our anxiety increases.

In order to help us focus on ourselves, we want to take inventory of our priorities and responsibilities. We need to recognize and remind ourselves that we are doing the best we can, rather than focusing on what others expect from us. Of course, there are still expectations of parents, caregivers, and teachers, and we still respect their expectations and work hard to understand their importance. At the same time, we need to stay focused on the fact that, while we will try to work hard, we are doing the best that we can, which means we may not always meet our parents', caregivers', or teachers' expectations, and that's okay, as long as we aren't behaving inappropriately or in destructive ways. It does not mean that we are not working hard or that we won't accomplish our set goals or meet those expectations all together. It doesn't mean that we don't care about their expectations or don't respect those who only want (or think they know) what's best for us. It does not mean that we won't be successful or that we are not good enough. (Here is where those core beliefs can influence how we perceive and interpret our experiences.) We need to be vigilant about our automatic thoughts and aware of the core beliefs that trigger our anxiety. We need to continue to evaluate those thoughts and practice shifting our focus to what we are able to do in the moment. This takes practice. Our way of thinking does not change overnight. We are essentially training our brain to think differently under stress than the way it typically has. Again, this takes practice.

When we are more focused on what others expect or want from us, we become less and less focused on who we feel we are, what is important to us, and what our own priorities or responsibilities are. It is critical that we are able to focus on ourselves and what is important to us, as opposed to what is important to others, because we need to develop our own sense of self. When so much of our focus is on others, we are not focusing on our own development. We can often feel lost or numb or not know what is important to us, what our passions are, or even what we want to do in our future. We want to help our kids learn how to focus on themselves at early ages. Yes, as I said before, kids will always work hard to please the adult figures in their lives, but we also want them to learn to recognize when it's important to focus on themselves in various circumstances, including with their peers.

As we respect the expectations of our parents or caregivers, parents also need to check themselves and let their kids make age-appropriate choices to develop problem-solving and accountability skills. It is natural for us, starting as young children, to work hard to please these important figures in our lives and make them proud. We want to live up to their expectations and make them happy.

However, as we become adolescents and young adults, we start to individuate from our parents and caretakers. This is a time when we are supposed to become more independent and think for ourselves, making more independent decisions, navigating social relationships and dynamics, and learning how to uphold our personal responsibilities. This does not mean that we no longer value what others want from us, but our focus needs to shift from doing things for others to doing what is right for ourselves. These choices that we make, whether they are good or bad, help shape who we are and our sense of self. We learn from these experiences. If we grow up consistently making decisions that we think others want us to make, even though those decisions may not be what we ultimately want or even what is necessarily in our best interests, we are not going to develop as strong a sense of self. In an effort to help individuate from our parents or caregivers, we want to try to stay focused on not just holding ourselves accountable for our choices and responsibilities but also working hard and doing the best we can in what we are working toward.

Anxiety and Its Relationship to Depression and Suicidal Thoughts

It is very common for those who suffer from anxiety to also suffer from symptoms of depression, which is the leading cause of disability in the United States in people ages fifteen through forty-four (Anxiety and Depression Association of America 2015; World Health Organization 2017). Suicide is one of the leading causes of death in the United States, and the second leading cause in people ages ten through thirty-four (National Institutes of Mental Health 2019; CDC 2017). According to the latest World Health Organization (WHO) estimate in 2017, more than three hundred million people are experiencing symptoms of depression, which is an increase of more than 18 percent between 2005 and 2015. The WHO speculates that the lack of support services for people who suffer from mental health problems combined with a stigma of mental health have been significant factors to preventing people from getting the treatment they need. This is where control theory can help destigmatize mental health and provide easy access and education, particularly within schools, to help decrease these numbers.

Understanding suicidal thoughts is critical; however, I'm not going to talk about crisis intervention. I want to emphasize the importance of how easy it is for someone to develop suicidal thoughts by way of anxiety and the overwhelming feeling of not having a sense of control in one's life. Suicidal thoughts should always be taken seriously. We want to be sure to understand the history of anxiety precipitating these thoughts and feelings and, therefore, be able to utilize objectives to manage and control the underlying anxiety, aiming to prevent suicidal ideations or the intent to act on these thoughts.

One misconception about anxiety and depression that I hear all the time, whether it be a presentation on mental health or stress management or even from other treatment providers, is that anxiety and depression are two separate things. Anxiety and depression are not separate or unrelated. Depression is actually a continuum of the anxiety scale. Depression results when we have already been battling high levels of anxiety for a prolonged period of time. When we find ourselves toward the top of the scale (around an 8, 9, or 10), it is extremely uncomfortable and overwhelming. We spend an exorbitant amount of energy—physically, mentally, and emotionally—when we are fighting high levels of anxiety. Although most people are not aware of what is happening with their anxiety and lack of control, we do know what it feels like to be completely overwhelmed.

We can't stay at the top of the scale for a prolonged period of time. We need to have some kind of relief on that scale. When we don't get a sense of relief and have been living at the top of the scale for a significant period of time, we eventually hit a wall, and we can't keep fighting the anxiety. To provide more context of this, think of drinking caffeine all day and all night. You are wide awake, going, going, going without any sleep. But we can't live without sleep. Eventually, our bodies are going to physically crash and burn. The same thing happens mentally when we are at the top of the scale for a prolonged period of time. We just can't live up there. We mentally crash and burn.

After being at the top of the scale for such a long time, week after week, month after month, year after year, the anxiety has physically, mentally, and emotionally wiped us out. We start to feel like we don't care about certain things anymore. We start to lose interest or pleasure in things we used to enjoy. We have no more motivation to keep doing what we've been doing on a daily basis. We feel like we just don't care. This is where depression comes into play. Depression is a continuum of the scale. We have been sitting at the top of the scale, fighting the anxiety day in and day out for weeks, months, or years on end, and we can't keep doing it. We are wiped out. We are completely overwhelmed. The anxiety has taken everything out of us. We feel like we've lost all control and don't know what to do anymore, and we don't see a way out of it. We feel helpless that we can do anything to make this feeling go away and feel hopeless that we will ever get out of this place. We've tried everything we possibly can to get out of this depression, and nothing has worked. We're helpless and hopeless.

Here is where we are highly vulnerable to engaging in self-destructive behaviors. We have been at the top of the scale for too long; we haven't had any relief; we are physically, mentally, and emotionally drained; and we don't know what to do. We've lost all control. We are desperate to find some kind of relief. What happens when we are in this state of depression for a significant period of time? We have tried everything we can possibly think of to get out of this depression, and nothing has worked. Again, we feel helpless and hopeless.

- We start to think, *Is this what my life is going to be like from here on out? This sucks.*
- We start to think about what it will be like to not live like this anymore.
- We think about the relief if we aren't here anymore.
- We think about what is wrong with us when everyone around us is so damn happy while we can't remember the last time we even smiled.
- We question if we are going to feel this way for the rest of our lives and, if so, can we actually live this way from here on out without experiencing any kind of positive emotion?
- We may think, *I would rather not wake up tomorrow than to feel this way for the rest of my life, but I don't see any way out of it.*

Are you starting to understand how someone may start to have suicidal thoughts?

Those who have serious thoughts of suicide, meaning that they have a plan and are intent on acting on this plan, are likely not going to tell anyone they have these thoughts or plans. I often see or hear that this is a myth about suicide; however, this is not a myth. If someone intends on acting on their plan, they don't want to be stopped. When someone speaks about having suicidal ideations, as much as we don't want them to feel this way or to have these thoughts, we want them to tell us that they have these thoughts. It's an indication that they feel stuck and helpless and don't know what to do. It's common to hear people say, after someone close to them has committed suicide, that they recently spoke to them and they seemed completely fine or happy. There was nothing to indicate that they were having a hard time. This is very common. It is not a myth. I've also experienced clients who have had intentions of acting on a plan and denied at the time of our session that they had suicidal thoughts or plans. Only after they came close to following through with their plan did they acknowledge what they had done.

I once spoke with an emergency room psychiatrist regarding one of my patients, who had been hospitalized for having suicidal ideations. Our patient had informed the psychiatrist that we were working on her anxiety, and the psychiatrist proceeded to tell me, "It's very rare to have someone with depression who also has anxiety."

The psychiatrist was treating anxiety and depression as two separate things and did not understand that depression is a direct result of anxiety. Someone who is depressed may not look particularly anxious because they have been experiencing heightened anxiety for a prolonged period of time to the point where they can't fight the overwhelming feeling anymore. At this point, the patient has already hit that wall where they feel completely wiped out physically, mentally, and emotionally. They are not necessarily going to present as being anxious.

This is a significant misunderstanding, by a psychiatrist no less, who does not understand how anxiety works. This is a problem. My client was not allowed to return to school until this psychiatrist approved of her going back. Yet the psychiatrist had no understanding of my patient's history of anxiety and how her anxiety affected her or even how she understood her own anxiety. He was strictly basing his diagnoses on how our patient was presenting at face value. Both the school and the psychiatrist failed to assess our patient accurately, and she was misdiagnosed in the hospital based on the psychiatrist's assumptions and his not understanding anxiety. I want to reiterate that this is a problem. We all need to be educated about anxiety and how it precipitates depression and suicidal thoughts. They are not unrelated.

When I'm working with clients who have reported feeling depressed or suicidal, my work is not focused on treating the depressive symptoms themselves. My focus is on addressing the root cause of the depressive symptoms, which is the anxiety. I will track the depressive symptoms and use them as mile markers because we obviously want the symptoms to decrease in frequency, intensity, and duration, but I'm not treating the actual symptoms. By tackling the root cause of the depression, the depressive symptoms will subside. If I strictly focus on treating the depressive symptoms and not treating the root cause of the depression, I will only be putting a Band-Aid over those symptoms. We can suppress certain symptoms, but if we aren't treating the cause of the symptoms, then the anxiety will manifest itself another way.

Think of the game Whac-A-Mole. When you hit one of the moles back into the hole, a mole will pop up somewhere else. Then you try to hit that mole, and another one pops up. The same thing happens with anxiety when it's not treated appropriately. We can work to eliminate certain symptoms of anxiety, but unless we understand what is causing the symptoms and get control over the core anxiety, we are just going to experience other symptoms of anxiety. If anger is one way in which our anxiety is manifested, we can consciously make an effort not to express our anger in such an aggressive manner, but again, if we're not addressing the root cause of our anger, we can start to develop a tic or start to experience gastrointestinal issues. No matter what the symptoms are, they won't completely go away if all we focus on is the symptoms themselves. If we treat the underlying cause of the symptoms, the anxiety, then the symptoms will actually start to subside.

According to the Centers for Disease Control and Prevention (2018), there has been a 30 percent increase in the suicide rate across the United States, averaging across all ages, since 1999. Furthermore, a study done by researchers at Yale University found that bullying victims are between two and nine times more likely to consider suicide than nonvictims (Yale University Study 2008). Unfortunately, the suggestions provided by the CDC to help prevent suicide are minimal. None of these suggestions include trying to understand what precipitates someone contemplating suicide. The listed warning signs presented by the CDC do not address the role of a person's sense of control, or lack thereof, and do not assess anxiety. Again, anxiety is severely misunderstood, misdiagnosed, and mistreated.

Neurobiology of Anxiety

As further evidence to show how anxiety affects our cognitive functioning and behaviors, Dr. William Stixrud, neuropsychologist and coauthor of *The Self-Driven Child*, has presented a neuropsychological model of what is happening in the brain when we are experiencing anxiety and chronic levels of stress. I will show how his neuropsychological model reinforces control theory. Dr. Stixrud recognizes that the National Scientific Council on the Developing Child identifies three types of stress:

1. Positive stress: This level of stress (anxiety) acts as a motivational factor for us to take the risks necessary to learn, grow, and work toward accomplishing short- or long-term goals. Applying control theory, an example of this level of stress may be when preparing for a test or competing at a sporting event. We may get nervous before the test or the event, but our anxiety can actually work to help us prepare ourselves as best we can by holding us accountable for studying or practicing our sport. (This is also where our anxiety can start to take too much control over us, where we can start to have thoughts or assumptions that we are going to fail or not perform well.) If our anxiety is not overwhelming or taking too much control over us and we are still able to maintain focus and concentration, we are going to be more likely to perform at an optimal level.

2. Tolerable stress: This level of stress (anxiety) occurs for relatively brief periods of time (not chronically), and we are

able to recover from this temporary anxiety. An example of this type of stress when applying control theory may be experiencing a loss, such as a breakup, a friend moving away, or even a death. Experiencing loss lowers our sense of control as we are not choosing for these losses to happen, and they personally affect us. These events are out of our control and are often unexpected. It may take some time for us to process these losses as we experience different emotions about these events. However, as we continue to process these losses, we eventually work our way to a place of acceptance. We may still be sad that these events happened, but we are better able to live with these changes in our lives.

3. Toxic stress: This level of stress and anxiety is chronic, lasting for longer periods of time or happening more frequently; is more difficult to recover from; and is a prolonged activation of the neurological stress system. Here is where we feel that such chronic stress is never-ending, or we don't see a way out. When applying control theory, this is when we have been experiencing a high level of anxiety for a prolonged period of time or have experienced a traumatic event (being abused, bullying, witnessing assault, being in an accident, etc.), and we feel we have (or have had for a period of time) zero control. We hit a wall, and we aren't able to effectively process such stressors anymore. We are physically, mentally, and emotionally wiped out. We don't have the energy to care or the motivation to do things anymore, and we experience the onset of depression.

As we remain in a state of depression, we start to feel more helpless and hopeless that there is a way out of this state. We have tried anything and everything we can think of, but nothing works. As Dr. Stixrud addresses, this is the level of stress that kids and adolescents often experience today. They have a difficult time managing daily pressures, such as getting the best grades, being compared to their peers, making sure they do enough community service for their college applications, taking AP classes in high school to bring up their GPAs, taking SAT prep classes, applying to the top colleges, playing sports or an instrument, participating in extracurricular activities, and the list goes on. This brings us back to the importance and main objective of control theory: to help students (and everyone) focus on themselves and what is in their own best interests, rather than taking on the expectations of others. As Dr. Stixrud indicates, this type of stress is debilitating for students and does not prepare them to manage their anxiety in the future. When students are focused on pleasing others, according to control theory, they are feeding their anxiety and not learning how to problem solve.

As previously mentioned, not all anxiety is bad. We need a healthy level of anxiety to motivate us to work hard and be successful in different areas of our lives. Dr. Stixrud also emphasizes the importance of optimal anxiety. The healthy level of anxiety that Dr. Stixrud refers to is short term or intermittent, and we are able to recover from this anxiety or stress and use it in a way that helps us be productive, focus, concentrate, and perform at a more optimal level. Self-care is important in aiding our recovery from anxiety.

Dr. Stixrud presents the neurobiology in a way that is parallel to control theory. He, too, emphasizes that control (or lack thereof) is at the root of our anxiety. Dr. Stixrud is able to explain more concretely what is happening in the brain when we undergo stress. The neurobiology that we will discuss includes the basic structure and function of the prefrontal cortex, amygdala, hippocampus, and pituitary and adrenal glands, as well as the role of the hormones dopamine and norepinephrine.

The prefrontal cortex is responsible for executive functioning. As previously mentioned, the prefrontal cortex is still under development during adolescent years. According to Dr. Stixrud, the prefrontal cortex doesn't stop developing until our mid-twenties, and our emotional regulation is not fully developed until our early thirties. As Dr. Stixrud explains, the prefrontal cortex is responsible for decision making, judgment, planning, and organizing and allows us to exercise control over our behaviors and choices.

The prefrontal cortex relies on two important neurotransmitters: dopamine and norepinephrine. When we experience mild stress, arousal, or excitement, according to Dr. Stixrud, the levels of these neurotransmitters increase just enough to where we are able to be more highly attuned to what we are doing in the moment. We are able to have clearer focus and concentration. However, when we experience higher levels of anxiety and stress or chronic or prolonged stress, our ability to focus, concentrate, and problem solve is compromised as the prefrontal cortex becomes overloaded with dopamine and norepinephrine. If we apply control theory, when we have been battling anxiety and have been toward the top of the scale for a prolonged period of time, it is much more difficult for us to focus on what we need to do in the moment and to problem solve. Our brains have been in overdrive and are flooded with dopamine and norepinephrine when we have not been able to recover or come down on the scale to experience some relief or a healthy sense of control.

In addition, Dr. Stixrud points out that when we have higher levels of these neurotransmitters working in our prefrontal cortex, we are much more vulnerable to making rash or impulsive decisions. This is also consistent with control theory, in that when we are at the top of the scale, we aren't necessarily aware of the fact that our anxiety is high and our sense of control is low, but we are highly aware that we don't like that feeling. If we are not aware of our anxiety or how we are interpreting information around us and don't like the way we are feeling but do not have proper tools to manage our anxiety and get back appropriate control, we are likely to engage in whatever is at our fingertips to help us feel better.

This is oftentimes impulsive and maladaptive behavior. We are less likely to think clearly or to identify appropriate options that are within our control to manage the stressful situation. We may feel better in the moment when we engage in these impulsive or maladaptive behaviors, bringing a temporary sense of relief or a false sense of control. But our actual sense of control stays low as we are not managing the root cause of the problem. Our anxiety will quickly return to a higher level, oftentimes worse than it was before.

Another aspect of the neurobiology behind anxiety, according to Dr. Stixrud, is what he refers to as the stress response system. This system is activated when presented with threatening information and consists of the amygdala, hypothalamus, hippocampus, and pituitary and adrenal glands. The amygdala is where our emotional processing takes place. According to Dr. Stixrud, the amygdala is sensitive to fear (which is a feeling of lacking control). He considers the amygdala our "threat detection system." Dr. Stixrud describes the amygdala as being reactive and "in charge" during high stress. When under high stress or high anxiety, the amygdala triggers our defensive behaviors, such as being reactive, aggressive, and inflexible.

This makes sense when applying the structure and function of the amygdala to control theory. When we are higher on the anxiety scale and our sense of control is low, we are more vulnerable to becoming reactive and defensive if our sense of control is threatened. This is also consistent with what we know about the function of the prefrontal cortex when under intense anxiety. We are more likely to make impulsive decisions and be more reactive when our sense of control is low and we are not able to adequately think through and focus on appropriate problem-solving objectives. It is a natural defense mechanism to feel on guard or protect ourselves when we feel threatened or a loss of control. Why won't we want to protect ourselves?

Unfortunately, our defenses can oftentimes be more harmful than helpful. That is why with control theory, along with cognitive-behavioral theory, we are trying to train our brains to think in a more logical step-by-step manner. We are teaching our brains to think differently than we have been used to thinking throughout our development and into adulthood. When we are able to think in a more logical, step-by-step manner, we are better able to focus on what we need to be doing in the moment and what our priorities are, identify options that are within our control, and problem solve more effectively.

The amygdala, being the emotional processing center of the brain, becomes more sensitive to fear- or anxiety-provoking information after we experience chronic stress. According to Dr. Stixrud, the amygdala becomes enlarged when we have been experiencing chronic stress, making us more vulnerable to reacting or experiencing heightened anxiety more frequently. As the amygdala becomes enlarged while the prefrontal cortex is compromised from chronic stress and anxiety, it becomes very difficult to distinguish between information that is actually threatening and information that is not, resulting in more generalized anxiety.

Let's get back to what is happening in the brain when we sense a threat. According to Dr. Stixrud, the amygdala sends a message to the hypothalamus and pituitary gland, which then send a message to the adrenal gland, which then secretes adrenaline. The adrenaline is a critical motivating factor to help us take action when under stress. All this happens subconsciously and instinctively. We don't think logically in high-stress or threatening situations. We react.

According to Dr. Stixrud, it is healthy to experience a quick, temporary increase in stress, as long as we are able to recover from it. This means that the hormones involved in the stress response are able to come back down, allowing us to experience some relief. In control theory, this is also considered a healthy increase in stress. If we are able to experience anxiety and learn how to manage stressful situations, we are learning how to exercise control over certain anxieties in a healthy way.

However, when we experience stress for a longer period of time, the adrenal gland secretes cortisol. According to Dr. Stixrud, when cortisol is released, it is more difficult for us to return to our baseline or recover from the stress. Chronically heightened levels of cortisol can actually "impair and eventually kill cells in the hippocampus" (Stixrud and Johnson 2018, 17), which activates and stores memories. Dr. Stixrud explains that this is why students often have a difficult time learning and retaining information when under stress.

Dr. Stixrud presents another great description of how the hippocampus works. Because it stores our memories, it is able to use these memories to help bring another frame of reference to our conscious awareness when we are experiencing a stressful situation. It helps us remember that we have had similar experiences before and were able to survive them or work through them, helping us calm down in the moment of high anxiety. He also puts this function into the context of those who have post-traumatic stress disorder (PTSD). When someone experiences extreme levels of stress or anxiety to the point of trauma, their neurotransmitters are overloaded, the stress-response system is activated, and cortisol is released, making it more difficult for the person to recover from the stress of the experience, thus damaging the hippocampus. If the hippocampus is damaged, the person is not able to recall useful information or memories of how to cope with stress. Dr. Stixrud refers to this as *perspective*. People with PTSD are not able to bring other perspectives to a new stressful situation that is in any way similar to a previous traumatic experience. They are not able to accurately put their current experience into proper context or recognize that it is not the same situation. They are highly vulnerable to experiencing a level of anxiety similar to what they experienced during the traumatic event.

Before we address the specific neurotransmitters that play a role in anxiety, let's go back to the role of maladaptive behaviors. Remember when we said that we are likely to engage in whatever is at our fingertips, including maladaptive behaviors, when our anxiety is high on the scale? If we know that smoking marijuana will help us feel better almost immediately and decrease our anxiety, then there is a pretty good chance that we will continue to utilize the same resource the next time we're feeling highly anxious. We may come down on the scale pretty quickly, but this will only last temporarily, and our actual level of control will stay very low. We're not doing anything to help manage the stressor that triggered our anxiety in the first place. We're going to keep going up and down on the scale, in a repetitive pattern, until we are able to break out of that cycle and find a more permanent way of managing our anxiety, ultimately gaining a greater, healthier, and more productive use of control.

Unfortunately, it can be very difficult to break this cycle. When we use marijuana, we feel better. It works. Why won't we continue to use it to help ourselves feel better? It's much easier than taking the time to work on raising our sense of control. When we find something that works, which brings our anxiety down and makes us feel good, we are at higher risk of continuing that behavior, even if it is not effective in the long run.

Now let's address what the neurotransmitters dopamine, norepinephrine, and serotonin do in this process. When we engage in a behavior that elicits a positive feeling, or what Dr. Stixrud refers to as a *reward*, the level of dopamine in our system increases. Higher levels of dopamine allow us to feel better and act as a motivator to engage in certain behaviors. We're going to be more motivated to engage in a certain behavior if we know it will make us feel better. Just as higher levels of dopamine are associated with increased drive, according to Dr. Stixrud, lower levels of dopamine are associated with lower drive or minimal motivation, as well as boredom. Dr. Stixrud states that there needs to be an optimal level of dopamine in order for there to be a healthy flow for optimal functioning.

What happens when we are under chronic stress? When we are experiencing prolonged anxiety, our dopamine, norepinephrine, and serotonin levels drop significantly. This makes it very difficult to do or want to do anything. In other words, according to control theory, here is where we hit a wall after experiencing prolonged anxiety, and we feel we can't keep fighting this overwhelming feeling. We start not to care about things. We feel a loss of motivation. This is where depression starts to come into play. We are physically, mentally, and emotionally drained. We just can't keep fighting the anxiety anymore. This happens when we have been experiencing chronic stress (prolonged anxiety). As Dr. Stixrud points out, this is the point where our dopamine levels drop significantly, and our motivation takes a major hit.

I hope that this information helps bring more perspective to understanding how the brain functions when we are experiencing anxiety. Dr. Stixrud provides an exceptional description of how these theories apply to kids in our current time, especially adolescents: "Chronically stressed kids routinely have their brains flooded with hormones that dull higher brain functions and stunt their emotional responses. Parts of the brain that are responsible for memory, reasoning, attention, judgment and emotional control are dampened and eventually damaged. Over time these areas can shrink, while the parts of the brain that detect threats grow larger" (Stixrud and Johnson 2018).

Furthermore, when our kids experience anxiety for extended periods of time, the prefrontal cortex is not able to develop the way it should. This is highly concerning, considering adolescents are too often experiencing higher levels of anxiety than adults and have a lower tolerance for stress than adults.

The objective here is to help ourselves and our kids understand our own anxiety and how to control it. We are teaching our kids tools that not only help them understand how to manage past stressors and manage stress in the moment but also increase their confidence so that they will be able to manage stressors that they come across in the future. Dr. Stixrud makes a perfect analogy: that by teaching our kids these skills and increasing our sense of awareness, we are in essence immunizing our kids. We are preparing them to know how to manage anxiety in the future, therefore, increasing their chances of succeeding in different areas of our life.

Screen Time

Another factor that affects our cognitive functioning is screen time. It's important to understand the extent to which screen time can impair the developing brain. Studies on screen time have consistently found that it has negative effects on the cognitive development of children, particularly those under the age of three. A study done by the US Department of Health and Human Services found that, on average, American children spend seven hours a day on electronic devices. (This includes television, iPads, iPods, smartphones, computers, and video games.) According to Dr. Aric Sigman at the British Psychological Society, screen time actually impedes a child's brain in developing specific abilities, such as focus, concentration, recognition of other people's tone of voice and emotions, communication, and even vocabulary building. This damage can potentially be permanent. Children under the age of three are in what is considered the critical period of the developing brain. The way in which a child's brain develops during the critical period affects how the brain continues to develop and function throughout the child's life (Margalit 2016). In other words, the critical period lays the foundation on which the child's brain continues to develop. Children need to be exposed to specific natural stimuli in order for their brains to develop healthily, specifically during the critical period. These natural stimuli need to come from the outside environment.

The stimuli that children need are not provided by electronic devices. By not getting the natural stimulation they need in order for their brains to grow, their development becomes stunted (Margalit 2016). Children need to learn how to process emotions and communicate with others, understand how others communicate with them, learn what different tones of voice mean, and even be able to visualize pictures and follow a storyline. When kids spend too much time on a screen, they are not using their own cognitive skills to figure things out. The device does the work for them, and they become lazy.

The frontal lobe, which is responsible for interpreting and comprehending social interactions, including facial expressions and tone of voice, is developed through "authentic human interaction" (Margalit 2016). The frontal lobe's most critical time of development is in early childhood. When kids have limited personal interactions because they spend excessive amounts of time in front of a screen, their emotional development and ability to read social cues can be stunted, potentially indefinitely.

Another important point that Margalit (2016) addresses is that when babies and children spend a significant amount of time in front of a screen, especially when they are using an interactive device, such as an iPad, smartphone, or video game, they become conditioned to receiving immediate gratification. Just as when adults engage in an activity that brings pleasure, as kids are able to swipe a screen to bring about new colors, images, and other stimuli, the neurotransmitter dopamine is released in the brain. Dopamine brings a feeling of pleasure and is a rewarding response. When children become used to this feeling of immediate gratification, they prefer this type of rewarding feeling to engaging in real interpersonal interactions. This behavior response is tantamount to behaviors in which adults engage, such as substance use, self-harm, and other risky behaviors, which help bring a temporary sense of relief or pleasure. In control theory, using electronic devices brings a false sense of control to children when they are conditioned to getting a desired response immediately and feeling an immediate sense of reward and pleasure.

According to Dr. Stixrud, every hour of screen time for a child is associated with increased blood pressure, while every hour of reading is associated with decreased blood pressure. He also states that the more technology kids use, the poorer their self-regulation is, and their executive functioning worsens. Self-regulation and executive functioning are twice as good at predicting academic performance success as IQ at all grade levels.

Anxiety and Its Relationship to Sleep

Sleep is one of the most critical factors, if not the most critical factor, in influencing anxiety. Sleep can directly affect a person's level of anxiety. According to Dr. Michael Breus and the National Sleep Foundation (2017), adolescents require between eight and ten hours of sleep per night, while adults require between seven and eight, and younger children need between ten and thirteen. When we don't get the amount of sleep we need, or a high quality of sleep, we are more vulnerable to experiencing higher levels of anxiety. According to Dr. Breus, research has found that only approximately 15 percent of adolescents are getting sufficient sleep. It is highly critical that adolescents receive consistent, quality sleep because their brains are still developing. They are highly vulnerable to experiencing health and safety issues and struggling with performance, focus, attention, ability to learn, information retention, and overall cognitive functioning when they are not getting their required sleep.

Sleep cycles for adolescents differ from those of adults and young children. Adolescents' hormones, particularly the hormone melatonin, shift to a later sleep-wake schedule and are triggered later in the evening than those of adults and younger children (Breus 2017). As a result, adolescents tend to naturally get tired and go to sleep later at night, closer to 11:00 p.m., while adults are more likely to fall asleep earlier. Therefore, adolescents tend to want to sleep later in the morning than adults. According to Breus, melatonin starts to work in the late afternoon for most adults; however, it has a delayed cycle with adolescents, and therefore, the melatonin level drops off earlier in the morning in adults than in adolescents.

The brain is very active even when we are sleeping. Sleep is when our body physically repairs itself, cleans out waste materials that can be harmful to our health, and processes and condenses emotional information (Breus 2017). Sleep is critical for the still-developing adolescent brain. The brain's prefrontal cortex is not fully developed and is the last part of the brain to reach full development. This is the part of the brain that is responsible for emotional regulation, decision making, and other executive functioning. Breus further supports that sleep deprivation in adolescents can lead to cognitive impairments, including the following:

- trouble with memory
- focus and concentration are diminished
- learning is impaired
- choices that are healthy and safe are difficult to make
- risk of engaging in risky behaviors as well as aggressive and impulsive behaviors and choices is increased
- judgment and decision making (and other psychosocial stressors) are poor
- emotional issues, including the following:
  o struggle with emotional regulation
  o irritability
  o generalized anxiety is increased
  o risk for depression and suicidal thoughts, social withdrawal, aggressiveness, and difficulty getting along with others is greater
- academic performance (including increased absences or tardiness) is a struggle

To highlight how important sleep is for our health, let's look at some research. A study conducted using lab rats found that rats died as quickly if they were prevented from sleeping as they did if prevented from eating (Lambert 2005). Other research found that sleep deprivation produces similar effects on the mind and body as chronic stress (McEwen and Karatsoreos 2015). This research also found increases in cortisol levels, reaction to stress, and blood pressure and decreased efficacy in the functioning of the parasympathetic nervous system, which is supposed to calm us. Sleep deprivation also produces inflammation, affects insulin production, decreases appetite, and depresses mood. This finding is consistent with control theory, in which a lack of sleep increases anxiety, therefore, decreasing our sense of control, focus, concentration, and self-regulation and increasing irritability.

There is no difference in performance on cognitive tests between older adolescents who sleep four to six hours per night for six weeks and those who don't get any sleep for three days. This study suggests that six hours of sleep or less is equivalent to chronic sleep deficiency. With sleep deficiency, the amygdala becomes more reactive in response to emotionally charged events, mimicking brain activity when experiencing high anxiety. This research is consistent with the neuropsychological theory of anxiety and control by Dr. Stixrud. These findings are also consistent with control theory. When we misinterpret information and make assumptions, we react more impulsively, decreasing our ability to think logically. We become more reactive than responsive. According to this study, our ability to see things in proper context is impaired, which then impairs our judgment.

Based on this information alone, it is evident how critical it is for children and adolescents to get the recommended (really required) amount of sleep. Students need to prioritize their sleep over staying up past what should be their natural bedtime doing their academic work. When students continuously sacrifice their sleep in an effort to complete their schoolwork, they are putting themselves at greater risk for more significant issues, as well as impeding proper brain development. These are both short- and long-term consequences, but this lack of sleep can ultimately have lifelong effects on physical, emotional, and mental health.

It is critical that schools, teachers, and the entire educational system take their students' sleep into account. The priority should not be on the amount of work placed on students. The priority needs to be on the health of the students. Without support for their needs and efforts to take care of their health, mental health, and sleep in particular, students will not be able to perform at an optimal level academically, physically, or even socially. If we are expecting our students to perform at their highest level at all times (which is an unrealistic expectation in and of itself), then we need to support their need for sleep and self-care. Furthermore, if students don't learn how to self-regulate (be aware of and monitor what their bodies and minds need), care for themselves, and manage their time effectively when they are adolescents, then we are setting them up for a lifelong struggle of anxiety and stress.

Continuing on the trajectory of minimal sleep and research findings, research from various sources has found a strong correlation between insufficient sleep and depression. Unfortunately, adolescents are more likely to use caffeine, nicotine, alcohol, or drugs to help manage their mood swings than to get sufficient sleep or learn appropriate ways to effectively manage their anxiety when they are tired. According to control theory, the less sleep we get, the more vulnerable we are to higher levels of anxiety, and the longer we are in a cycle of restricted sleep and increased anxiety. Eventually, we hit a wall and feel we can't keep battling the anxiety anymore. We start to experience symptoms of depression when we hit that wall. Competitive academics are not worth jeopardizing brain development or emotional regulation. It puts young people at a higher risk of developing anxiety and depression while simultaneously diminishing their sense of self-worth. These are long-term, potentially life-altering effects just to finish an assignment that has no bearing on how successful a student will be throughout their life.

Another study that Dr. Stixrud references involved two groups of sixth graders. One group was asked to sleep one hour more than usual for three nights, while the other group was asked to sleep one hour less than usual for three nights. The study found that students who had as little as thirty-five minutes less sleep than the others performed at a fourth-grade level on cognitive tests, effectively losing two years of cognitive ability (Sadeh et al. 2003). According to Dr.

Stixrud, numerous studies have found a correlation between weaker academic performance and self-reported decreased sleep time. There are also studies of more than nine thousand students showing decreases in absences and tardiness, more alertness in school, and improved mood (which means a decrease in anxiety) in schools that have later start times (Wahlstrom 2002).

So how do you work with your child when they aren't prioritizing their sleep? Here are some guidelines:

- Start by presenting a choice: You can choose to go to bed at a reasonable time (demonstrating responsibility), and you will be able to perform better in school tomorrow (as well as feel better, feel less anxious, be able to more effectively manage stress, etc.). If you choose not to go to sleep at a reasonable time, you are choosing to make yourself more vulnerable to feeling anxious and not being able to focus, concentrate, or perform at the level you need or want. If your performance and grades are important to you, I hope you choose to make sleep a priority in order to do your best.

- Promote winding down in the evening, creating a routine to help your child fall asleep or get into sleep mode. For example, stop any screen time (phones, television, computer, video games, iPads, etc.) about one hour before bedtime. Have them do a quiet activity (reading, taking a shower, meditation, listening to music, etc.).

- Have them do screen-time homework earlier in the evening.

- Encourage tech-free zones in the house.

- Foster a consistent bedtime for every age.

- Have them abstain from any caffeine, which can trigger anxiety itself as well as interfere with their sleep cycle.

- Use light exposure in the morning to help reset their circadian clock and reestablish an appropriate sleep-wake cycle.

Defense Mechanisms

What happens when we are not aware of anxiety or don't know appropriate ways to help ourselves feel better in those moments of stress? When we are not aware of our anxiety or how it is affecting us in the moment, we are likely to become defensive. We are more likely to react impulsively or irrationally or engage in some kind of avoidant behavior. Our defenses are natural reactions when we feel threatened, when things don't go the way we want, or under any circumstance, when we feel a lack of control. It's our body's natural fight-or-flight response. We try to tackle the situation at hand by exercising control, albeit often in inappropriate or maladaptive ways, or we often avoid dealing with the anxiety-provoking situation. Using the scale from 0 to 10, when our anxiety is higher on the scale, around an 8, 9, or 10, we tend to have a very difficult time focusing, concentrating, or thinking rationally. Because we have a harder time thinking clearly when our anxiety is higher, we are more vulnerable to engaging in maladaptive behaviors that tend to be more impulsive or provide us with an immediate sense of relief, particularly when we are not aware of our anxiety and, therefore, do not know how to control it in a healthy manner. Even if we do not understand our anxiety, we know how we feel when we are at the top of the scale. We are well aware of the fact that we do not feel good and that it's too much to handle. At this point, if we are not aware of appropriate or healthy ways to help ourselves feel better when consumed with overwhelming anxiety, we are going to look for whatever is at our fingertips to help us feel better. More often than not, we will engage in maladaptive behavior. These maladaptive behaviors, which are outlined below, help bring an immediate sense of relief. Our anxiety goes down on the scale. While these maladaptive behaviors only bring temporary relief or a false sense of control, we still choose to engage in them for a time-out from the anxiety, rather than sit with that overwhelming feeling with no relief in sight.

We can see a pattern of losing control or not having the level of control or sense of safety or security that we need when we look at significant life-altering experiences. These significant or traumatic life experiences can form negative core beliefs, especially in those of younger ages, making them more vulnerable to living with a heightened level of anxiety throughout their development and into adulthood. These experiences may include, but are not limited to the following:

- Experiencing loss
- Being bullied
- Being abused verbally, physically, or sexually
- Being neglected physically or emotionally
- Witnessing abuse of any kind
- Experiencing racism
- Not feeling they are living up to others' expectations
- Feeling like a failure
- Experiencing divorce or having parents going through a divorce
- Losing a home due to various circumstances
- Constantly being compared to others
- Feeling unnoticed or not validated
- Having an alcoholic parent
- Having a family member in jail
- Being involved in the juvenile justice system
- Experiencing abandonment or forced separation
- Being in foster care
- Witnessing violence
- Experiencing war
- Seeking asylum

Unfortunately, these examples are only a handful of the significant life events that people can experience. However, all these situations are examples of when a person has limited to no sense of control. These are circumstances that are thrust upon them by someone or something else. No one chooses to be put in these situations. It's not just the actual events that can have a significant impact on a person; the way in which the person interprets or experiences an event can be additionally damaging. This becomes the mental narrative of their life and their view of themselves in their life story. For example, a child may assume that they are unlovable or a burden on their family or others, and that's why they are abused. They may internalize the belief that they deserve to be abused and don't deserve to be treated any differently in future relationships.

Loss is a significant example in which there is a substantial drop in our personal sense of control, whether it be death, a divorce, and personal trauma, such as losing a house in a fire or flood or losing a pet. These are all examples of significant loss that we do not choose to have happen. Unfortunately, we are left with trying to figure out how to get to a point of acceptance, after having emotionally processed our significant loss, and learning how to move forward in our lives. We have to learn what we can do for ourselves moving forward by focusing on the options that are within our control. Grieving helps us move through this process. We initially experience a state of denial, where we logically understand what has happened, but it is too much for us to emotionally process right away. Our brain needs time to think through and process the event, eventually making way for us to emotionally process that loss. Our emotions are all over the place, going through feelings of denial, anger, bargaining, and depression before finally getting to a place of acceptance.

According to the CDC (2018), a study that collected data from 2011 to 2012 found that children who were currently experiencing anxiety or depression were more likely than those not experiencing depression to have one or more of the following:

- another mental, behavioral, or developmental disorder, such as ADHD, a learning disability, or speech or language problems
- other chronic health conditions
- school problems
- parents who reported high levels of stress (their own anxiety) and frustration with parenting
- unmet medical and mental health needs

If a child is experiencing any of these issues, where is their sense of control likely to be? Their sense of control is going to be lower when they are not receiving support or care for medical or mental health issues. Their sense of control is going to be lower when they have parents who have high anxiety and unpredictable behavior. Their sense of control is going to be lower when they don't know how to successfully manage school problems or when they have a learning disorder, making it difficult for them to understand the material. When kids have a hard time understanding, sustaining attention, or listening, they are not going to feel they have a good sense of control in those circumstances, making them vulnerable to assuming negative thoughts about themselves that they aren't smart, will always be less than others, are a failure, etc. Chronic health problems prevent kids from being able to engage in routine daily activities, again limiting what they can do and their sense of control.

See a pattern here? It's understandable that if a child is struggling to learn material in school in the same capacity as other students, they are not going to feel they have control over their learning or academics if they are not able to meet the same expectations as their peers. This then leads students to start to feel like they aren't smart, or at least not as smart as their classmates, and they start to internalize these negative beliefs about themselves, affecting their core beliefs and self-esteem. If a child doesn't know how to get the support they need, again, they are not going to feel like they have control over their stressor.

Understanding Avoidance

Avoidance is one of the most common natural defense mechanisms. It's our flight defense mechanism. It makes sense. Why would we want to face an anxiety-provoking situation if we don't have to, right? Avoidance will alleviate our anxiety in the moment, but it's only temporary, similar to other defense mechanisms or maladaptive behaviors. It is not a means of exercising control in a healthy or effective manner; rather, it provides a false sense of control. The anxiety will eventually increase again, oftentimes becoming higher than it was initially, and our sense of control stays very low on the scale. We don't actually gain control over the situation when we avoid it, and we then anticipate having to avoid it in the future. Until we understand why we feel anxious, confront the stressor, and identify what we can do to get some sense of control back, the anxiety will remain. When we avoid, we are putting off having to deal with the stressor, but that anxiety will still linger until we feel we have a greater sense of real power to change the situation.

Unfortunately, it is much easier to avoid a stressor in the moment than to confront the situation. When we are forced to deal with a provoking situation, we are likely to automatically assume the worst is going to happen and feel that we don't have the level of control we want or need in the moment. If we feel that we have everything under control and that things are happening predictably or as planned, then we will not be experiencing high anxiety. However, in the moment of stress and not feeling like we have full ability to shape a situation's outcome, we are prone to assume that we won't know what to do or how to handle the situation. It can be difficult to focus in the moment or shift our focus to what is within our control.

When our anxiety is high on the scale and we are feeling extremely overwhelmed, avoidant behaviors can quickly bring some relief to that uncomfortable feeling. We can quickly lower our anxiety on the scale by avoiding an anxiety-provoking situation, whether it is happening in the moment or we are anticipating having to deal with a stressful situation. For example, if a student experiences high anxiety when at school, it's common for them to try to avoid going to school. They may feel sick (not just claim to be sick but actually feel sick as a symptom of anxiety). They may experience anxiety or panic attacks when going to school or even thinking about going to school. If students are not educated about anxiety and taught to identify options that are within their control to appropriately and effectively manage the stressful situation at school, they are likely to engage in avoidant behaviors.

As students avoid school, it becomes harder for them to return. The longer they avoid it, the worse the anxiety gets. They start to become more dependent on their avoidance of school in an effort to manage their anxiety; however, they aren't getting any actual control over their anxiety. A student will likely feel temporary relief from their anxiety when they make the decision to skip school that day, but that anxiety is likely to return later that evening when the student knows they have to return to school the next day or the next morning when they are waking up or getting ready for school. Although some students may be well aware of why they don't want to go to school, they often don't know how to manage the stressor that is triggering their tension or fear. If they don't know what to do to manage the stressor—be it a test, a bully, social stressors, etc.—they are not going to feel they have a good sense of control, which heightens their anxiety, making them want to avoid the situation altogether and retreat to their comfort zone or safe space.

Oftentimes, schools will have a tutor come to the student's home when they have not been able to return to school. But having a tutor come to the student's home is actually enabling the student's avoidant behavior and essentially increasing their anxiety. The student is not learning how to appropriately manage their anxiety and regain control and confidence. They are not learning how to manage the stressors at school that are triggering their anxiety. They are allowing these stressors to have control over them. The next time they experience similar events, they are not going to know what to do or how to handle the situation. Their immediate response when presented with similar circumstances is likely to avoid the situation and default to their cop-out solution. Until they understand their anxiety and learn appropriate ways to manage it and understand how to gain control over the stressor, their anxiety will continue to return, inhibiting their ability to engage in various situations or perform in more optimal ways.

Another example of avoidance as a defensive reaction is behaviors stemming from a fear of abandonment. Recall from our discussion about core beliefs that if a child is placed in the care of another who is not their initial caretaker, especially if they have already established a firm attachment with their initial caregiver, the child may then anticipate being abandoned by other caretakers or by others with whom they try to establish a relationship throughout their development and adulthood. It is common for a child who has experienced people coming into their lives and then leaving at some point to assume that they will be abandoned by others. They are likely to have a difficult time allowing themselves to fully engage in a relationship (romantic, friendship, or otherwise) without anticipating the other person leaving them. The child, even as they develop into adulthood, is likely to push people away or detach themselves if they feel they are getting too close to someone and will be hurt by losing that person. When the child creates a barrier with another person, preventing them from getting emotionally close to that person, the child is able to exercise a sense of control to prevent getting hurt again. In other words, they can avoid experiencing another personal reaction and loss of their own sense of control.

Lastly, let's review the example from earlier in the book about Katie, my client who was able to recognize that her panic attack was caused by hearing the word *suicide* in one of her classes, even though the attack didn't occur until the end of the day when she was sitting down, relaxing. This is also an example of how avoiding processing an anxiety-provoking event, intentional avoidance or not, does not relieve the stress. Until we can understand the source and, therefore, identify what we can do that's within our control, we cannot manage anxiety-provoking situations. Coping skills will only help alleviate our anxiety temporarily. They won't prevent the anxiety from continuing to affect us, and we aren't finding the source of the anxiety by just using coping skills. These skills can help calm us when our anxiety is high on the scale, but once we've come down to where we can think more logically, we need to utilize cognitive objectives to address the cause of the anxiety, giving us more insight and, therefore, a better understanding of how to control it. As previously stated, when we avoid having to deal with the stressor, that anxiety will linger until we feel we have a greater sense of control over the situation.

Substance Use and Self-Harm

Substance use is another example of avoidant behavior. When our anxiety is high on the scale and we are feeling overwhelmed, we are going to look for the fastest and easiest way to alleviate our anxiety if we don't have the awareness or education on ways to exercise healthy control.

Let's go back to the example of a student experiencing high anxiety at school. Avoiding school may or may not be the primary choice to alleviate the student's anxiety. Students may choose alternate routes to avoid dealing with their stressors. If alcohol and drugs are easily accessible, there's a good chance that students will think about using substances. If they choose to use drugs or alcohol when feeling highly anxious or stressed, they will feel their anxiety decrease rather quickly.

Unfortunately, drugs and alcohol do often work in the short term. If we have a drink or two or more, we can numb uncomfortable feelings. We can bring ourselves down on the anxiety scale and feel a temporary sense of relief. We may actually feel pseudohappy for a short amount of time, feeling a false sense of control. If we smoke marijuana, our anxiety will go down. If we take some prescription pills, we can try to numb our worries. Self-harm, such as cutting, can also bring that quick sense of relief by distracting us from our emotional pain with physical sensations. It makes sense. All these actions will give us some kind of relief through diversion. They are ways to avoid emotionally processing and managing anxiety.

What happens when that temporary relief starts to go away? Our anxiety goes right back up on the scale, oftentimes worse than it was before we engaged in the maladaptive behavior. The next time we start to feel that overwhelming anxiety again and we don't have the proper tools or awareness to know how to manage it, we are going to use what worked before, again, and again, and again. It works, right? So why won't we do it again?

Here is where we get caught in a trap where our anxiety comes down temporarily when we find something that works to alleviate that awful feeling, but then the anxiety soon returns to the higher level on the scale. We get trapped in a cycle of dependence on the maladaptive behavior that helped bring us relief, even if it was temporary. Our anxiety keeps going up and down on the scale but staying lower for increasingly short periods of time in a downward spiral. We become dependent on these maladaptive behaviors to help us feel better when we don't have adequate awareness about our anxiety and don't know appropriate ways in which we can control it. However, the relief becomes less effective over time and with repeated use of this crutch, as the problems of the real world are banging down the door. You can't avoid them forever.

But that's just it—it's temporary. The use of a substance or self-destructive behavior will only temporarily bring relief from the anxiety, bringing us a false sense of control. Our actual level of control is still minimal. We are not gaining any control over the anxiety or overwhelming feelings by depending on a substance to alleviate that awful feeling. But because it works, usually very quickly, and this is all we know to alleviate the anxiety, we are at risk of developing a dependence on a substance or a behavior in an effort to manage our overwhelming anxiety. We have not gained any control over our anxiety (or the source of the anxiety) by engaging in these behaviors. We may feel like we are on top of the world for a bit, but then we start to feel powerless, desperate, and disgusted with ourselves. The root cause of that anxiety still needs to be identified and addressed.

Other Avoidant Behaviors

Other avoidant behaviors that we may experience or witness are lying, manipulating, blaming others for our actions, and justifying or making excuses for our wrongful actions or choices. These avoidant behaviors are examples of not taking accountability for our decisions.

Lying

An example of lying as an avoidant defense mechanism is if a child, Jimmy, hits a friend, Thomas; and Thomas runs to his parents to tell them what Jimmy did. Jimmy will quickly feel an increase in his anxiety. Granted, children are typically not aware of anxiety, nor do they understand this abstract concept. However, they are well aware of their uncomfortable feelings even if they can't verbalize them. If Jimmy is afraid of getting in trouble, his anxiety is going to be higher on the scale. Usually, kids don't like to get in trouble. If Jimmy is anticipating that he will get in trouble (an example of an automatic thought without having evidence it will happen), then Jimmy may assume his parents will be very angry with him. If his parents are angry with him, he won't be able to keep playing, he will have to go to his room, he will miss out on something or not be able to play with Thomas or his other friends, his friends will think he's not a good kid, they will make fun of him, and on and on. His thoughts will spiral.

What does a child do when he's consumed by these automatic thoughts? Naturally, he will likely go into defense mode. He's thinking of the fastest solution to prevent getting in trouble or upsetting his parents. The first thing Jimmy may think of in that moment is to lie to his parents and say he didn't hit Thomas. He may think that if he lies, he will avoid getting in trouble. He will avoid the embarrassment of admitting he acted inappropriately. Let's say Jimmy lies to his parents, and his parents believe his lie. In that moment, Jimmy's anxiety drops dramatically on the scale. He feels a big sense of relief because he avoids getting in trouble. He avoids his parents getting mad at him. He avoids losing playtime or time with his friends. He avoids being embarrassed. He also avoids taking personal responsibility for his actions. What does Jimmy learn from that experience? If he's afraid of getting in trouble in the future, he can lie again so he doesn't get in trouble. He doesn't learn how to take accountability. If lying works for him, there's a good chance that he's going to do it again if he's in a stressful situation where he is being held accountable for something and doesn't want to get in trouble.

If we don't learn how to take ownership of our actions when we are younger, we will continue to engage in the same maladaptive behaviors or find other avoidant maladaptive behaviors to use each time our anxiety spikes as we continue throughout our development and even into adulthood. If our immediate gut reaction is to lie or place blame on others throughout our development and we aren't taught about the importance of accountability, then, as adults, we are going to do the same thing. We need to teach our children appropriate and healthy ways to manage stressful situations, especially when we are at fault, or their actions will translate to real-world issues. Furthermore, parents need to react appropriately so their kids aren't scared to tell the truth and to communicate that lying may be worse than the actual behavior.

Now let's think about what these defense mechanisms turn into as we get older. What do these behaviors look like in adults when we aren't taught how to appropriately manage our anxieties? Adults who never learn how to take accountability for their actions are likely to justify their behaviors (to themselves and to others), make excuses for why they did what they did, blame others for their mistakes, or manipulate others to do what they want or take the blame. They will experience temporary relief of anxiety in the moment if they can blame someone else or justify their actions, convincing themselves that what they did isn't really that bad or that they themselves are really not at fault. But they know what they did is not right, and they will continue to lie to cover previous lies or work even harder to convince others that they aren't wrong. This sounds stressful and tiring.

Let's go back to the example of Jimmy and Thomas. Why did Jimmy hit Thomas in the first place? What was the purpose of that behavior? It might have been his way of trying to control Thomas. Jimmy might not have liked the fact that he wasn't getting what he wanted from Thomas.

When we engage in aggressive behaviors, it is often a defensive response. We may be trying to get something we want or to exercise control over others in order to get them to do what we want. We are also struggling to accept that we don't have control of what is happening in that circumstance or that we don't have control over another person. We don't want to accept that we are not getting what we want. When we have a hard time accepting that we don't have control over others or various circumstances, we often try to exert control in other ways or up the ante and put pressure on others to get what we want. This leads us to our next topic: manipulation.

Manipulation

Manipulation is another example of how we act in order to exert control over others to try and get what we want. It's common to engage in manipulative behavior when our anxiety is high and we don't want to accept what is not within our control or take account-ability for our own actions. If a child wants something, such as a toy that another child is playing with, they may or may not understand that they have to wait their turn. Also, kids often do not want to wait their turn. They also don't like to hear the word *no*. When they are told no or that they can't have what they want, they are going to up the ante in order to get what they want. They may yell, bite, hit, etc. Kids have a hard time accepting what is not within their control because, in many cases, they don't have much control. They want what they want when they want it. If they can't get what they want, they try whatever it takes to convince others to give them what they want.

Kids are master manipulators. It's a natural defense mechanism for them as they are trying to figure things out in the world. They are trying to learn what they are able to do, what they can't do, and what they're not allowed to do. Manipulation is part of a child's develop-ment. They will come up with every possible reason that they should be allowed to have what they want. They just don't want to accept the answer no. Again, kids do not like to accept what is not within their control. When they are not getting what they want, they quickly become frustrated or angry. In other words, they become anxious. They feel anxious in that moment when they aren't getting what they want. Although kids don't exercise this level of conscious, abstract thinking, they are no less prone to reacting, often in inappropriate ways, when they don't have the level of control that they want or need.

Another way in which kids can manipulate us to get what they want is by splitting their parents. Oftentimes, kids will ask one parent for something, and when that parent says no, they will go ask the other parent. The child (usually) won't mention that they already asked the other parent. They will just try a new tactic with the second parent.

Here's an example from when I was about eight years old. My parents owned a business in our town, and right around the corner from our family's business was a grocery store. I was hanging out at our business one day and went over to the grocery store. In front of the grocery store were some girls with a box of puppies, giving the puppies away. I really wanted a puppy. My mom came over to the store. (I'm not sure if she was actually looking for me, but let's pretend she was.) She saw me with the puppies. I asked her if we could have one. She said no. Now, my parents are animal lovers, and we already had a dog, so I really didn't think it was a big deal as a kid. I started to beg and plead. She told me to go ask my dad. "If your dad says yes, then I'll say yes."

I was so excited. I brought a puppy over to my dad at work and asked him if we could keep it. He asked me what my mom said. I told him, "She said yes!" I purposely left out the part where she said, "If your dad says yes." I remember thinking that I wasn't being totally honest, but in my mind, I wasn't completely lying either. I was justifying my actions and what I told my dad in my head. Since my dad was under the impression that my mom had already made the decision and said yes, he said yes.

I ran back to the store to find my mom and told her that my dad said yes. (He did!) Later that night, when my parents were home, I found out that they had a discussion about the dog. I'm not sure how the conversation went exactly, but it was along these lines:

"I didn't say she could have a dog."
"She said you said yes."
"I didn't say yes. I said I'd say yes if you said yes."

"Well, she told me that you said yes."

So in summary, I didn't like the first answer I got from my mom, I upped the ante and guilted her, I manipulated my parents and our conversations, they didn't communicate with each other in the meantime, and I got a new puppy. I found a way to get what I wanted.

There are exceptions for babies or children with special needs when reacting to various situations when their behaviors aren't necessarily manipulative. Babies will cry when they are hungry, tired, or in pain. They aren't being manipulative, but they are communicating that their needs are not entirely met, and they are not happy. Essentially, they don't have the level of control they need in a particular situation, albeit in a more primitive form. However, as they get older, we still have to set limits with them and communicate to them in a such a way that they understand that they are not always going to get what they want, such as watching television all day or eating cookies whenever they want. We have to start teaching them about the word *no* very early to facilitate their ability to accept when they are told no throughout their development.

Children with special needs may also escalate their behaviors if they feel their needs are not being met or if they are feeling completely overwhelmed or overstimulated in their environment. They may not be trying to manipulate a situation when their behavior escalates physically, but they are still communicating that they don't feel in control, and it's too much. They need help communicating effectively when they don't have the skills to do so yet, and we need to be mindful of this. Communication (which will be further discussed later in the reading) is key for each and every person to feel they have a greater sense of control.

Violence and Aggression

Another defense mechanism can be manifested through aggressive or bullying behaviors. Bullying and aggressive behaviors are additional examples of how we can exercise a temporary (false) control when we feel we don't have the desired level of control in one or more aspects of our lives. It's much easier to project our anxiety onto others, make others feel less about themselves, and put our and others' attention onto others than to focus on ourselves and take accountability for our own behaviors. If we don't have a strong or positive sense of self, resulting from high anxiety, it's easier to exercise control over others than to acknowledge how we feel about ourselves. We don't want to acknowledge our vulnerabilities because we will likely interpret these vulnerabilities as weaknesses. Instead of focusing on what we need to do to take care of ourselves or take accountability for our actions and choices, we can more easily exercise control over others and project our anxiety onto them. Therefore, we don't need to focus on ourselves. We convince ourselves that we're not the ones who are struggling, but it's everyone else who has the problem. They become scapegoats.

We are more likely to engage in violent or aggressive behaviors when we have already been battling high levels of anxiety for a prolonged period of time, meaning we have been feeling a loss of control, or limited control, for a significant period of time. We are at the top of the scale, having little to no relief on the scale and very little, if any, sense of control over significant areas of our lives. As previously discussed, when we are at the top of the scale for so long with no alleviation from the stress, we eventually hit a wall where we physically, mentally, and emotionally can't keep fighting the anxiety. We eventually start to feel helpless and hopeless after we try numerous things to help us feel better and nothing works. It feels like this awful feeling will never end. This is also where depression comes into play, as mentioned earlier. We become desperate for control and want to end our suffering.

An example of this level of aggression and violence is mass shootings. The decision to engage in such a violent way is likely not an impulsive decision or reaction. We need to think about what warning signs there might be that can result in someone feeling the need to exert power over others to such a degree. What might that person have experienced where they continuously felt a loss of personal control? In addition to the previous list of life circumstances that limit our sense of control, we need to ask these important questions:

- Were they bullied as a child or throughout their development?
- Did they feel they weren't living up to others' expectations?
- Did they feel like a failure?
- Did they feel they were constantly compared to others?
- Were they feeling unnoticed or not validated?

When we have been experiencing these circumstances, especially over a prolonged period of time, the anxiety wipes us out, and we fall into a state of depression, leading to a state of helplessness and hopelessness. Not that we don't need to hold individuals accountable for creating mass destruction, but we also need to consider what precipitates a person acting in these ways, to empathize with them, and to understand how to help others who can potentially be in this state of despair. This doesn't mean we need to agree with the choices they make, and again, they need to be held accountable for their actions, but people don't get to this level of destruction for no reason. We need to get to the root of these patterns and educate those around us, especially our children and students, so we can all learn why we feel anxiety, where it comes from, and what our anxiety does to us and learn healthy ways of exercising control rather than engaging in maladaptive and destructive behaviors. (I will further address bullying when discussing communication.)

Aggression and violence are ways to avoid reflecting on our own needs and vulnerabilities. It's easier to justify to ourselves that others are responsible for where we are today and why we are struggling. However, here is where we want to work on identifying our automatic thoughts and shift our focus to what we can do for ourselves moving forward. For example, if we experienced being abused as children, we want to focus on where the power of control is. When we were children, our abusers exercised control over us. However, after recognizing this, we are able to work on shifting that control back into our own hands, where we can hold our abusers accountable for their actions and what they did to us while recognizing that we are taking back our control. We can also hold others accountable if we ever feel taken advantage of or controlled. We need to know that we are in control of ourselves and not allow others to have control over us.

Fear of Rejection and Loss

Another significant factor that tends to precipitate avoidant behaviors is the fear of rejection. Most people do not want to feel rejected in any aspect of their lives. It's a painful and embarrassing feeling. Where is our sense of control when we experience rejection? It's very low. We feel we have a limited sense of control in circumstances where we feel vulnerable and rejected. Think about what is happening when we are rejected—another person is making a decision that affects us. We are not making that decision ourselves. Someone else is making a decision for us. It's not within our control, yet we have to accept the decision that is being made. If we are the ones making the decision, we will have control and, therefore, will not feel rejected. No one wants to be rejected. We all want to be the ones shaping our own destiny and making the decisions, but that's not the reality in every situation.

Examples of when we may anticipate rejection include someone for whom we have feelings; family members leaving; us moving between foster homes; and us being rejected by a school we wanted to attend, a job for which we interviewed, or a social group. Ultimately, we don't like when situations do not go the way we would like, especially when we feel our selves are being deemed not worthy of love, inclusion, acceptance, etc. Separation anxiety and fear of abandonment are examples of when a child anticipates losing or being separated from a significant attachment figure in their life. When a child is fearful of losing an important person in their life, the child does not feel confident that that person will always be in their life, and their sense of personal control over that relationship is minimized.

Unfortunately, rejection can have a lasting effect on us. Our assumptions can easily take complete control over our minds, and we quickly start thinking of the worst-case scenario when anticipating being in a vulnerable position. Rejection can also be difficult to accept when that early experience of rejection is so significant that it results in our internalizing negative core beliefs about ourselves.

Young children are constantly trying to live up to the expectations of their parents, caregivers, teachers, etc. They are very focused on what others think and feel about them. They want to please others and do what makes others happy and to feel that others approve of them. Unfortunately, this can come at a cost. It's good that kids try to do well by others, don't get me wrong, but they often become so focused on what others think of them that it becomes all-consuming, and this mindset can impede a child's ability to focus on themselves. For example, a child, Evan, experiences a situation in which he makes a bad choice or even makes a genuine mistake, such as spilling his milk at the dinner table, and his parents react by saying, "Evan! Why did you do that? I can't believe you just spilled your milk! Why can't you pay attention?"

Evan can easily interpret his parents' reaction to mean that he disappointed them and feels or assumes that his parents won't love him in the way they used to. He may continue to assume that he will always be a disappointment to his parents and may, therefore, anticipate his parents rejecting him in some way or not approving of him. Evan's parents may not verbalize anything about being disappointed in him, but based on how they reacted in the moment when Evan made a mistake, he could easily interpret that experience as being a disappointment to his parents.

Another example is if a child, Susie, feels she doesn't get as much attention as her brother, she may feel rejected. Susie may assume that there is something wrong with her or, similar to Evan, that she is unlikable or unlovable and that she doesn't deserve attention or any kind of special treatment. Kids want to please their parents or caregivers and will often do whatever they can to make them proud. They may feel that if they are able to please their caregiver, maybe their caregiver won't reject them, at least not in that moment. Kids will often try to please others in order to feel accepted. They become more concerned about upsetting others, not fitting in with others, and being rejected than they are about themselves and what they feel is in their own best interests. As previously discussed, these assumptions can easily be internalized, essentially becoming part of the child's core beliefs. The child can also generalize these beliefs to other aspects of their life throughout their development or assume that if they disappoint their parent once or twice, that they will always be disappointing their parent or others.

Another example is if Charlie doesn't get invited to Jake's birthday party, knowing that a lot of his friends are invited. He can very easily assume that Jake doesn't like him, that he has done something to make Jake mad and not invite him, or that other kids don't want him there. He may also start to compare himself to his peers, thinking or assuming that he isn't as much fun as the other kids, he's not as likable, he's not as smart, etc. It is very hard for kids to focus on themselves or recognize what is actually true when faced with stressful social situations. Charlie struggles to recognize that if he didn't do anything wrong, then it's on Jake (or Jake's parents) as to why he isn't invited, and he shouldn't feel bad about himself.

Because kids don't always verbalize what they are thinking or feeling, these negative and personal assumptions can easily become rooted as core beliefs if they are not addressed. These core beliefs will then continue to trigger anxiety as we get older. If Charlie continues to believe that he is not well liked by others as he gets older, he will likely assume or anticipate not being invited to other parties or social gatherings, generalizing this assumption to be true of any future social engagement. He may avoid engaging with others if he anticipates being rejected in any way and continues to internalize that he is unlikable or that others don't want to be around him. These core beliefs will then easily trigger anxiety in other areas of his life, such as when he tries out for a sports team or a play or applies to college or for a job. He may assume that he is not going to make the team or land a role in the play, that he isn't going to get accepted into the schools of his choice, or that an employer won't want to hire him because he is not a likable person. Even if Charlie has worked hard throughout his schooling or career and has applied himself to the best of his potential, he will more likely focus on the negative core beliefs instead of recognizing his other strengths and qualities. He will have a difficult time not comparing himself to others and will assume that no matter the circumstance, he will continue to be unlikable, potentially limiting himself in taking risks, applying for jobs, or pursuing new relationships or friendships.

So how do we deal with rejection and manage potential rejection? Here is where we want to identify any automatic thoughts that are triggering our anxiety. We need to identify what we are afraid of happening, anything that we are anticipating or assuming to be true. We then want to review these thoughts to see if there is any evidence that these thoughts are absolutely true.

- Do I know for a fact that I'm definitely not going to get the job for which I applied?
- Do I know for a fact that I'm not a likable person and that others don't like spending time with me?
- Do I have proof that if I don't make the team, it's because the coach doesn't like me and doesn't want me on the team?
- Do I know for a fact that I'm not capable of becoming a decent ballplayer or that I won't be able to learn and succeed at a new job?
- Do I have proof that I have been a bad friend to make others not like me?

Where is the evidence? Kids can't do this themselves; they need a parent to reassure them of their inherent worthiness.

If we don't have proof to show that any of our automatic thoughts are true or that they are definitely going to happen, then we need to practice shifting our focus to what we know to be true and what is currently happening. We want to shift our focus to what we know we're capable of doing and what we've already been able to accomplish (providing evidence against our assumptions) and, most importantly, focus on ourselves. We do not want to compare ourselves to others. Comparing ourselves to others can make us more vulnerable to thinking and internalizing negative thoughts about ourselves.

Once again, when we compare ourselves to others, we are essentially giving others our control. We are allowing others to influence how we feel, what we do, and how we act. We are not focused on ourselves and what we need to be doing that's in our own best interest. When we are able to focus on ourselves, we shift that control back into our own hands. We want to continue focusing on our own strengths and skills, reiterating what we are capable of accomplishing as well as the evidence that shows we have already been able to succeed in various areas of our lives.

It is important for us to work hard and identify personal goals for ourselves, reflecting growth in areas we value. For example, we still need to work hard in school or apply ourselves as best we can to do well at work. But we also need to stay focused on our own strengths and skills rather than comparing ourselves to others. When we start comparing ourselves to others, we become vulnerable to assuming negative thoughts about ourselves or feeling that we aren't as good or as smart enough as others around us. It is also our choice which areas we want to master. We don't have to play baseball or join a band because we think it's cool or because that's what we think others want us to do. We can pursue what is meaningful to us. It's our choice and no one else's. Sometimes people find themselves trying to win a race they don't even want to run.

For example, even if I don't get the job for which I applied, I know that I can still be successful at another job or in the same field. That job, or not getting hired for a job, does not define what I'm capable of attaining. If I don't do well on the SATs, that doesn't mean that I won't get accepted into a good school or be successful in my future. If I can stay focused on what I know I can do and continue to hold myself accountable for my own responsibilities, knowing that I'm doing my best, then I will be more capable of accepting that I didn't get into the school of my choice. I know that I'm a good student. I work hard, I'm dedicated, and I take school and work seriously; all of which gives me more evidence that I can and will be successful in school and work because I know what I'm capable of accomplishing. I'm not going to let a test score, a school, or a job determine if I will be successful. They do not define me. Rejection does not define me. Granted, it is still important to take accountability for the things I need to work on, improve my skills, and accept and utilize constructive feedback, but I also need to stay focused on the fact that I'm choosing to hold myself accountable for these areas of progress and know that I can still be successful in what I pursue. I'm the one defining who I am and what I can accomplish. I have the control.

Regarding relationships, if we're anticipating being rejected by someone for whom we have feelings, we should try to stay focused on what we ourselves are capable of providing in a relationship. If someone chooses to not be with us from the outset, and we did nothing to hurt this person (at least not intentionally), then we need to recognize that it is their choice to not engage in the relationship. However, their decision does not indicate that we are not engaging, that no one will want to be with us, or that we won't be able to establish and maintain healthy and successful relationships. It is their own personal choice, which is separate from who we are.

We also have to accept that we can't control another person and convince them to be with us. We need to stay focused on who we are, independent of the other person. Furthermore, if that other person chooses not to be with us, we need to be mindful that we don't give that person control over us to the point where we change who we are to meet their needs or please them in ways that are not true to ourselves. We want to know that we are presenting our real selves, and if other people choose not to engage with us, that's their choice. Again, we need to practice shifting the focus back to ourselves, review the strengths and qualities we have independently, and not let that rejection define us or take away from our own sense of control.

We can also experience rejection after having been in a relationship for a significant period of time. Let's face it—not all relationships are lasting, yet no one wants to feel rejected by their significant other. In this case, we still want to focus on ourselves and our role in the relationship. If we know that we have done everything we can to try to make the relationship work, such as actively communicating and listening to and supporting the other person to the extent that we can, then we have done the best we can. However, we have to recognize that we are not independently responsible for making the relationship work; the other person is equally responsible.

On the other hand, if we have done something that hurts the other person in the relationship, we need to take accountability for our actions. Our partner may or may not forgive us, but if we take full ownership of our choices and understand what we need to work on moving forward, then we are following through with our responsibilities in the relationship. We can't undo what we have done, but we can take accountability for the choices we have made and the choices we make moving forward. If our partner then chooses to end the relationship, even after we have taken full ownership of our actions, then at least we know that we have done what we can after the fact. This means we have managed the situation as best we can, but we need to accept our partner's decision to end the relationship. Our focus should then be on the fact that we have taken accountability for our actions and have done the best we can to mend the relationship, the things we learned, and the things we can do moving forward in our future relationships.

A study conducted at Duke University (Psychology Today 2017, 55) used a scale that measured the extent to which people would go in order to be accepted by others. Although it is beneficial to feel a sense of belonging in some capacity, that longing to belong to a group can also come at a cost. Dr. Mark Leary of Duke University stated of their research that "People who are higher in the need to belong may have greater problems saying no because of concerns about rejection. They also might have a strong fear of negative evaluations, so they worry that saying no will cause others to judge them unfavorably. People are concerned about the disappointment, frustration, or inconvenience that their refusal might cause" (Flora 2017). I have found this to be very common in my own clinical work.

It can be costly to our sense of self when we are highly focused on what others want, how to please others, how to meet others' expectations, or how not to upset anyone. If we say no to someone when taking into account what we need to do for ourselves or what is in our best interests, and the other person becomes angry or upset, we can validate their feelings and let them know that our intention is not to upset them but that we have to do what's right for ourselves, even if the other person does not agree. It is the other person's job to accept that they don't have control over others and that situations are not always going to turn out the way they want. Others are not always going to do what we want or agree with us all the time, and we have to learn to accept that fact. We are not responsible for managing their feelings, just as they are not responsible for managing ours.

Even in instances when we are willing to help others and do what is asked of us (specifically when it is not interfering with our taking care of our own responsibilities), it does not mean that the other person decides how and when we do things. We are still able to have a say in how we help others; for example, "I would be happy to help you move into your new apartment, but I won't be able to stay all day. I can come in the morning or even help you pack, but I have to be back home by a certain time to take care of other responsibilities." We can create boundaries so others don't walk all over us. I will address boundaries to a greater extent in the discussion of communication.

One last example comes to mind with regard to rejection. I came across a story on National Public Radio's *All Things Considered* (2017) about a gentleman named Christian Picciolini, who is the founder of a group called Life After Hate. Christian is a former white nationalist who spoke out about the violence in Charlottesville, Virginia, in August 2017. He provides an example of how people, particularly young people, have a need to belong and to feel accepted. Being accepted into a group is often a way to prevent feeling rejected and, in this case, a vehicle to become violent. Christian has been working to reform white nationalists through his organization. He makes a very valid point, saying, "I think ultimately people become extremists not necessarily because of the ideology. I think that the ideology is simply a vehicle to be violent. I believe that people become radicalized, or extremist, because they are searching for three very fundamental human needs: identity, community, and a sense of purpose." He goes on to talk about experiencing abandonment when he was younger, which led him to this community. (This is also very similar to how others can become involved in gangs.) He states that a lot of younger people often feel lost and don't have a lot of hope and end up searching for "very simple black-and-white answers."

I feel this example speaks directly to the point of control theory, in that it is very easy for us to allow others to exercise control over us (whether it's intentional or not) when we don't have a strong sense of self or self-esteem. If our self-esteem is low and we don't have a strong sense of who we are individually, our anxiety is automatically high. It's very easy for us, especially as children or adolescents, to follow what others do or to make decisions that we feel will win the approval or acceptance of others. Once again, we give our control to others rather than being responsible for ourselves. We aren't focused on who we are as individuals or what is important to us personally. Our focus is on what we think others want of us, and we make decisions that please others rather than those that are in our own best interests. It is very easy to lose our sense of self and self-control when our driving forces are a fear of rejection and the need to belong. This provides another example of why it is so critical for us as adults and parents to teach our kids healthy ways to exercise control and strengthen their personal sense of worth through learning responsibility and accountability.

Communication

How do we work with others in an effective way, even if things aren't going the way we want? How do we get others to understand our perspectives, thoughts, worries, or concerns? How do we work with kids to help them learn how to make better choices and not act aggressively when they don't get what they want? How do we help kids stop others from bullying them? The answer: communication. The focus: control. When we communicate, we are exercising healthy and productive control, as well as helping establish a healthy sense of control for our kids. When used appropriately, communication is one of our most significant tools for exercising control and managing our anxiety. The following communication objectives can be applied to both kids and adults.

Validation, Setting Limits, and Providing Choices

Adriana is told to stop playing and clean up her toys because it's time to eat dinner. Adriana doesn't want to stop playing and doesn't do what she's told. Her mother continues to tell her to clean up, and Adriana continues not to listen or to do what she is told. Her mother's frustration (anxiety) increases as she feels Adriana is not listening to her. When a parent feels their child is not listening to them, they aren't going to feel like they have control over the situation; hence, the anxiety quickly increases.

While trying to convince Adriana that she needs to clean up, her mother may raise her voice as she's getting frustrated, which will increase Adriana's anxiety. By raising her voice, her mother is using a maladaptive approach to control Adriana and get her to do what she's told. If Adriana is being told to do something she doesn't want to do, her mother's frustration or anxiety increases as she feels she does not have the level of control that she wants in that moment, and Adriana will also feel as though she is being controlled to a greater extent as her mother continues to raise her voice.

How does the mother communicate with Adriana to get control of the situation? If Adriana starts to get upset because she doesn't want to stop playing, her mom can validate her feelings by letting her know that she understands Adriana doesn't want to stop playing, and she's allowed to feel mad that she has to clean up, but then set a limit by giving Adriana a choice. She can choose to do what she's told and clean up her mess so there won't be any consequences, or if she chooses not to listen and not to clean up, then her mother will take her toys away or she will lose playtime after dinner. The mother can validate her daughter's feelings, present the two options, and then ask, "What's your choice?" When her feelings are validated, Adriana's frustration or anxiety will likely start to come down even slightly because she is given the message that it's okay to feel upset, and there is nothing wrong with that feeling, even though it's not comfortable. Adriana will also feel like her mother is listening to her if her feelings are validated. Just like adults, when kids feel like they are listened to, their sense of control will increase, which automatically starts to decrease their anxiety. By providing Adriana with choices, her mother is setting boundaries and letting Adriana know that Mom is in charge, and Adriana can't always do what she wants. Adriana, therefore, learns how to accept when things don't go her way.

Parents need to be consistent with setting limits and following through in order for their child to learn how to accept when they don't have control over something and that not everything will go their way. At the same time, by giving the kids choices, they are still able to exercise control and decide how they want to handle the situation. Adriana can still make a good choice and not have a consequence. By asking Adriana, "What's your choice?" her mother transfers responsibility from the parent to the child. The question reiterates that it's Adriana's choice and her responsibility to handle the situation appropriately. If Adriana chooses not to make a good choice, she will essentially learn that she is accountable for her own actions and choice. The choice being made is not the mother's (and the mother doesn't want Adriana to get a negative consequence), but if Adriana decides to make a wrong choice, then she learns accountability (again, with consistency from her mother setting limits). The mother can reiterate that Adriana made the choice not to clean up and, therefore, chose to have a consequence. It was not the mother's choice. Her mother can also reinforce that she has Adriana's best interest at heart and wants her to learn to recognize her responsibility in her decisions.

There is still a benefit to a child making the wrong choice as they start to learn the importance of accountability. Accountability is another significant tool to help decrease anxiety. As Adriana learns about accountability, she will also experience a decrease in her anxiety. Because she's taking ownership of her behaviors and choices, she learns to accept when she doesn't get her way and when she doesn't have control over a particular circumstance. Furthermore, by providing Adriana with choices, the mother exercises control over her own anxiety by not getting into a power struggle with her daughter. By transferring responsibility to Adriana, she is giving her daughter an opportunity to exercise control while still setting boundaries for her. Both Adriana and her mother are able to maintain control of their anxiety and have a better, healthier sense of control by communicating rather than engaging in an argument.

What happens when we don't communicate effectively? Think about when you are trying to talk to someone and they talk over you or they aren't paying attention. Do you feel like they are listening to you? Do you feel like you have control in the conversation when the other person isn't listening to you? If we don't feel we have control, our anxiety (frustration, anger, and annoyance) automatically increases. What do we tend to do if someone isn't listening to us? We may raise our voices, or we may interrupt them. We do this as a reaction to not feeling the level of control we need in that moment. We are trying to exercise control over the other person; however, raising our voices or talking over them is not actually going to give us control. We will feel more of a false sense of control. In that moment, if we raise our voices, our anxiety may come down just slightly on the scale, but our actual sense of control stays very low. Our anxiety will quickly return to a higher level on the scale the second the other person raises their voice or interrupts us again. What starts to happen is that we get into a power struggle. If we raise our voices over the other person, they will likely do the same, and we keep getting louder and louder, interrupting each other and not listening to what the other is saying. We are both fighting for control, yet the conversation turns into an argument, and neither one of us has control. In fact, our sense of control keeps lowering the more we argue, which automatically increases our anxiety.

How do we maintain or exercise appropriate control in a stressful conversation? First, we need to practice listening. We may not necessarily like what we hear all the time, but we need to listen to others. By practicing listening, we are allowing the other person to communicate more effectively, even if they are more emotional in what they are saying. The person speaking is going to feel they have at least some control in the conversation if the other person is listening.

Once that person is done presenting what they have to say, they will likely allow us to have that same opportunity to express our concerns. This also teaches us to accept when others may not agree with us (accepting what is not within our control). Keep in mind, just because we are working on communicating effectively and appropriately, it does not mean that we always have to agree with the other person or have the same opinion or perspective. We are focusing strictly on the way in which we communicate.

Now, if we feel that another person is talking in a rude, inappropriate, or disrespectful way, we can still exercise appropriate control by setting a limit with that person: "If you continue to be disrespectful to me, I'm not going to engage in this conversation. If you choose to speak and act respectfully, then I will listen. It's up to you." This is an example of how we can set a limit and hold the other person accountable while maintaining appropriate control at the same time. We are not controlling the other person. We are giving them the message that we will not allow them to speak to us disrespectfully, that they don't have control over us, and that we are not doormats. If they still choose to be disrespectful, we can say, "You've made your choice. I'm not going to continue with this conversation. You can let me know when you are ready to have an appropriate conversation."

We can then walk away. We maintain control of ourselves. We don't allow the other person to have control over us. We hold the other person accountable while still allowing them an opportunity to resume the conversation if they choose to act appropriately. The more consistent we are with setting limits, holding others accountable, and following through with these limits, the more others will start to understand what to expect from us. They will understand that they can't control or manipulate us, but we won't shut them out either. They will understand that we are still willing to work with and talk with them, if they approach us respectfully.

Once each person has had an opportunity to present their concerns, we want to make sure that we understand each other. This is where we validate, or repeat back to the other person, what they have said or how we understand they feel. When we receive validation, we again feel like the other person is listening to us, even if they don't agree with us. The main point is to listen and understand the other person's perspective. Again, we don't have to agree with them, but it is important to understand their perspective. If we repeat back to the other person what we understand from what they have said and have completely misunderstood them, they then have an opportunity to correct us and clarify what they have said.

This is an important step. If I'm listening to someone and I misinterpret what they are saying, I can very easily start to assume they mean something else, and my assumptions (automatic thoughts) will start snowballing, and then I'm jumping to conclusions, getting more and more frustrated (anxious). As I'm creating all these false assumptions in my head, I'm becoming more vulnerable to reacting irrationally and losing my temper and my sense of control. I can nip this reaction in the bud if I simply repeat back to the person what I think they have said. If I'm wrong, they can correct me and, therefore, prevent me from creating more assumptions in my head and losing control in the conversation. Keep in mind, it's our responsibility to communicate our assumptions or understanding of what was said to the other person.

This communication approach is effective for people of all ages. We can use these objectives when talking with other adults, teenagers, and even toddlers. Think about how toddlers react when they don't feel understood. We see more aggressive behaviors and meltdowns. As they learn how to communicate better and more effectively, those negative behaviors tend to decrease because they learn other ways to communicate where they feel they have more control. If we can teach our kids these communication tools, they will likely be able to communicate much more effectively throughout their development and as adults. They will be able to handle social situations more effectively. They will be able to set limits with others and hold others accountable when needed. These positive techniques and objectives are transferred to adulthood. If children are taught accountability when they are younger, they will be more likely to take accountability for their actions as they get older and will, therefore, be able to manage their anxiety more effectively and be better skilled in relationships and many domains of life.

Self-Control

An example of how our children learn the importance of self-control is in the home. When a child is raised in a chaotic environment with limited structure or rules, they don't experience having a solid sense of control. When they are in a chaotic environment, they feel chaotic, just as a game without rules is chaos—the rules give the game meaning. At the other end of the spectrum, when kids are in a highly controlled environment with limited ability to explore and learn on their own, they will feel controlled, and their anxiety is already heightened. They are highly vulnerable to experiencing anxiety. They are likely not taught to self-regulate in a healthy manner and are less likely to have tools to help calm them. These environments increase the risk of kids engaging in defensive or maladaptive behaviors as a primary coping mechanism to alleviate their anxiety. They experience a lack of containment, which essentially inhibits their ability to feel safe.

We need to have a middle ground. When children are provided structure, routine, and rules, even if they don't like the rules, there is a feeling of safety and comfort. This safety comes from having a predictable routine with understandable rules and consequences, teaching them accountability and teaching them to accept that they don't have control over everything or over others, that not everything goes their way, and that it's okay. If a child's environment is predictable, they are going to have a stronger sense of control and a better understanding of their own responsibilities. When anxiety is not dealt with at a young age, it then continues into adolescence and adulthood, where children tend to have a higher baseline level of anxiety (although they are unaware of it) and have a hard time self-regulating, communicating, or even creating their own daily or weekly structured routine, let alone managing their anxiety effectively.

Bullying

Another example of how kids can utilize these interpersonal skills is when they are bullied. When a child is taught interpersonal or communication skills, they will be more prepared when another child tries to overpower or emotionally damage them. We want our kids to know how to maintain their own sense of self and self-control. We want them to understand that no other kids can control them, while, at the same time, they can't control other kids. They are in control of themselves.

If a child is being bullied, we want them to know that they can set a limit with the bully or aggressor and hold them accountable. Initially, if a child is being bullied, their anxiety is going to quickly increase. They will (we hope only momentarily) feel a loss in control when another child is overpowering them and trying to control them through physical violence, humiliation, ostracism, or other emotional abuse or manipulation. When a child experiences this power dynamic, we want them to be able to recognize it. We want them to have a fundamental understanding that it is not okay for others to control them in an aggressive or manipulative way.

One of the most important words we can teach our kids is *no*. When a child is being bullied, we want their automatic response to be "No!" This is one of the most important limits that a child can set. Just by telling their aggressor no, they are giving the bully the message that the bully cannot control them. They are telling the bully that they are in control of themselves and do not have to do what the bully tells them to do or allow the bully to make them feel bad about themselves in any way. We need to teach our children the importance of this word, not just for protecting themselves but also in the context that if we choose not to respect someone else telling us no, we are choosing to have the consequences.

Kids, as well as adults, need to understand how critical the word *no* is, no matter the circumstance. Kids need to learn that they cannot control other kids or intentionally hurt them or make them feel bad without repercussions. If they choose to act in any of these ways, they will be held accountable, and there will be consequences for those actions. The word *no* also teaches kids about accepting what is not in their control. We all have to understand that we can't have control over everything or over other people. What we do have control over is ourselves and the way in which we can communicate in order to get things done, get the help we need, or hold others accountable.

Although the word *no* has power to it, there is oftentimes a concern as to why people often struggle to say no. People often fear how others will react. We fear that we will be humiliated or that others will seek retaliation if we say no to them or hold them accountable in any way. We need to understand that it is critical for us to hold others accountable and to say no to them when they are crossing boundaries and harming others for the sake of getting what they want. We need to be able to focus on the fact that others are not entitled to have control over us in negative, harmful or threatening ways. We are in control of ourselves, whether others like it or not.

When we don't say no to others and do not hold them accountable, we are allowing others to have control over us. We are giving them the message that what they are doing is okay. Even if we are anticipating how that person may react if we set a limit with them (although we don't have proof that they will definitely react in a negative way), we still need to set limits and hold them accountable. Again, if we are consistent in setting limits, eventually, others will know what to expect from us. They can't have control over us. When we stop ourselves from setting limits because we are afraid of how the other person may react, we are giving them our control. Consistency in limit setting is critical.

There will still be times when saying no to someone may not work. This is actually typical when we haven't previously been setting limits with others and we have (unintentionally) allowed others to overpower us in some capacity. When we start setting limits, what often happens is that the other person doesn't like the shift in control. When we set limits, we are giving them the message that they no longer have control over us and that we are in control of ourselves. This is often difficult for the aggressor to accept, at least initially. In addition to being consistent with setting limits and holding the bully accountable for their behavior, we can present a choice to them if they continue to not accept no as an answer: "If you choose not to respect my answer and continue disrespecting me, you are ultimately choosing to get a higher authority involved. That's not my choice. That's the choice you are making as you choose to continue these inappropriate behaviors."

You are not threatening the other person but are pointing out the fact that the situation will reach another level if they choose to continue acting in an aggressive manner. You are continuing to hold the person accountable by putting the responsibility for their behaviors on them. You are not going to take responsibility for their behaviors or continue to allow them to exercise control over you.

I started working with Shawn during the spring of his junior year in high school. Shawn was a very talented, smart, and responsible young man. He was a very strong student, was active in several sports, was hardworking (he even earned his Eagle Scout Badge), and had many friends and some very good close friends. Shawn had always been respectful of others, had always had good relationships with his teachers and coaches, and had very strong relationships with his parents and sister. I started seeing Shawn when he was having a hard time with two of his then friends inside and outside of school. These were friends who Shawn had known since elementary school. They had been inseparable up until high school. As they started going through high school, Shawn became friends with other classmates but still remained good friends with his two buddies from childhood. He wouldn't exclude them to do anything but rather tried to include everyone when getting together. Over the course of a couple of years, Shawn's two friends started to treat Shawn disrespectfully. They would publicly humiliate him and also took their behavior to social media. But that wasn't enough. They went on to blackmail Shawn in order to have control over him. As strong as Shawn was, he's also human and has a breaking point. He had become overwhelmingly anxious over the course of two years, to the point where he was significantly depressed. He was still able to go through his days, meeting his responsibilities, but the depression took hold of him. He was at a breaking point. This was when he started coming to therapy.

My work with Shawn focused on anxiety management. I didn't treat his depressive symptoms. I explained what anxiety is and that it is rooted in experiencing a lack of control. We took a deeper look into the ways in which his "friends" were exercising control over him. For whatever reason, they wanted to hurt him, emotionally. They wanted to cause him pain. They wanted to humiliate him. We didn't know why they behaved in these ways or why they were out to get Shawn, but there was a good chance that they were struggling with their own sense of self and self-esteem. It was possible they were jealous of Shawn.

We also talked about if there was anything Shawn might have done to upset or frustrate them, but we weren't able to identify anything, which was consistent with his character. Shawn was able to give examples of when he was messed up and was able to take accountability for his actions. He didn't struggle to take ownership in his choices. This was an area I immediately explored with my clients. However, I did not find this to be an area of concern for Shawn. Given that he truly felt he did not do anything (at least intentionally) to hurt his friends, we shifted our focus to identify ways in which

Shawn could start to take control back over his life and not allow others to have that hold on him anymore. We focused on the fact that his "friends" didn't have control over him, but that he had control over himself. We focused on communicating and setting limits with others that allowed Shawn to feel a greater sense of personal control, while letting others know that they couldn't have control over him. We practiced holding others accountable for their behaviors and choices. We reiterated over and over again that they did not have control over Shawn, but that he had control over himself.

Shawn started to lay out choices for these two classmates. He let them know that if they chose to continue to threaten him, then they were choosing to get school authorities involved and were ultimately choosing to be given natural consequences for their choices. He let them know that they were choosing to lose a longtime friend and would continue to lose friends if they kept treating others the way they had treated Shawn. Shawn put the responsibility on them. He worked hard to take his control back. Shawn continuously held them accountable any time they started to cross a boundary, which reinstated every time that they did not control Shawn. He was in control of himself.

Within a matter of three months, Shawn gained tremendous insight to his own anxiety, as well as how it affected others, and was able to bring his anxiety levels down significantly. Because he tackled his anxiety, his depressive symptoms subsided. He was happy again. All this work happened before the school year ended.

Fast-forward to the fall of Shawn's senior year in high school. Shawn was on the football team. He was still in the locker room after practice one night, after most of his teammates left. There was one other teammate, an underclassman, sitting on the bench with his head down, crying. Shawn sat down next to him and asked what was wrong. His teammate opened up to Shawn and told him that he was being bullied. Shawn quickly empathized with him and told his teammate his own story. Shawn also told him that these other kids didn't have control over him. He emphasized to his teammate that no one else had control over him and that he was in control of himself. Shawn continued to tell his teammate what he did to get his own personal control back when he was bullied. The key work he emphasized was control.

Later that evening, Shawn's mother received a phone call from that teammate's mother, thanking her and Shawn. It turned out that the student who was crying on the locker room bench was planning on taking his own life that night. After Shawn took the time to sit and talk with him and he heard what Shawn had to say, he decided not to follow through with his plan.

Imagine being told that: You have helped save another student's life. Or your own child has helped save another student's life. The word *powerful* isn't strong enough to describe what happened. Imagine if we bring this education into schools where everyone can work together to lift each other up and, who knows, save each other.

One other important example of understanding the word *no* is with regard to sexual harassment and assault. If we teach kids when they are young that they don't have control over others, and vice versa, as they get older, we can instill the message that control also refers to assaulting others. We want our kids to learn how to hold others accountable and continue to practice this throughout their lives. We want to help them be prepared to focus on ways in which they are in control and to hold others accountable for their actions if someone tries to exercise inappropriate control over them. In addition, we want our adolescents, young adults, and children to understand that they are not allowed to exercise harmful and inappropriate control over others and that they, too, will be held accountable for their actions. If they practice setting limits and holding others accountable for unhealthy or inappropriate choices, others around them will start to see this pattern and will know what to expect from our kids: that if someone chooses to control them inappropriately, they will be held accountable and will have consequences.

Enabling versus Taking Accountability

Accountability is one of the most crucial objectives we need to focus on and practice, as well as teach our children and students. When we learn to take accountability for our actions, we are actually taking a significant step toward lowering our anxiety and increasing our overall sense of control.

What Does It Mean to Take Accountability?

Taking accountability means that we are taking complete ownership of our behaviors, choices, and roles. We will specifically be referring to taking accountability under stressful circumstances. When we take accountability, we are not blaming others for our choices or behaviors. We are not justifying our actions or making excuses for ourselves. We recognize that we are independently responsible for our actions and the role we play in situations that cause ourselves or others harm or discomfort or result in putting ourselves or others at some kind of risk.

When we take ownership of our choices and behaviors, we are better able to recognize how our decisions and actions affect other people. We are more likely to reflect on how we will respond to a situation if someone else makes the decision we have made. We are better able to take into account others' perspectives and understand how others want to be treated.

When we are in a situation that requires us to take accountability for our actions—for example, when we make a mistake at work, forget to do something, or have to cancel on someone—our anxiety is naturally going to go higher on the scale, and our sense of control will drop. If we don't feel like a situation has played out the way that it is supposed to and if we recognize that we have made a mistake or canceled plans on someone and put them in a difficult situation, we are likely to feel some type of anxiety. We don't feel we have the level of control that we need or want when situations don't turn out the way we have planned. In order to bring our anxiety back down on the scale and our sense of control up, we need to take accountability for our actions. We need to recognize that our actions and choices can have a negative outcome, whether it affects us personally or affects others in a negative way. Unfortunately, we can't undo what we have already done. However, we want to manage the situation as best we can by taking accountability for our actions or choices. We need to recognize that we have made the choice; no one else has made that choice for us.

As we are able to take full ownership of our choices or mistakes, our anxiety will immediately start to decrease, which automatically starts to increase our sense of control. We are doing exactly what we should if we happen to make a mistake or make the wrong choice. We are bound to make mistakes and wrong choices from time to time. After all, we are human. But we want to shift our focus from the fact that we have made a mistake to how we handle the situation moving forward. If we make a mistake at work, what will our supervisor want to see? Do you think they want to hear excuses? Do they want to hear us justify our actions? What if we blame others for our actions? They don't want to hear it. All they want is to hear us take accountability for our actions. They will be more accepting of our mistakes if we take ownership of them. They don't want to hear excuses from their employees. They want to know how we are going to handle the situation moving forward. This is the message we want our kids to learn—that it's okay if we make mistakes, and the important thing is how we manage our mistakes moving forward, which includes telling the truth. If we teach our kids early how to take accountability, we are setting them up to more successfully manage their anxiety throughout their lives and to gain maturity and the respect of others.

When we start to make excuses, justify, or blame others for our decisions and actions, we are not taking accountability for our behaviors. Doing any of these will cause our anxiety to come down on the scale in that moment, giving us a false sense of control. However, that relief of anxiety is only temporary. Our anxiety will quickly return to a higher level on the scale when we don't take accountability for our actions. In that moment, we are convincing ourselves that what we have done is okay and justified, but our actual level of control stays low because we are not taking the proper steps to appropriately manage the situation.

When we do take accountability, again, our sense of control will increase because we aren't trying to hide what we have done, justify, make excuses, or blame anyone else for our actions or choices. We are likely to understand what we have done, how it is our own independent choice, what we need to do differently, and how to manage the situation moving forward. As we take accountability for our actions, there is likely to be a slight increase in anxiety prior to acknowledging our mistake. However, that anxiety will quickly come down once we admit what we've done. If we know what we need to pay attention to moving forward or what we need to do differently, we are increasing our level of control, therefore, decreasing our anxiety.

If we think about being in a situation where someone else makes a mistake, how do we feel if they give us an excuse or justify why they did what they did? How do we feel if they blame someone else (or us) for their actions or decisions? What happens to our anxiety level on the scale? It's likely to increase. For myself, I will feel very frustrated if someone was making excuses for their behavior and not taking accountability or acknowledging that what they did was not a good choice. However, if that person takes responsibility for their actions and acknowledge how their choice affects others, my frustration or anxiety will go down on the scale. I will feel an increased sense of control because I won't feel I have to convince that person that what they have done is wrong. If I feel they understand what they have done and are not making excuses, fully accepting that the choice is theirs, and understanding what they need to do moving forward, I will feel like the situation is managed appropriately and there is nothing more I need to do. Not only will the person who has made the mistake bring their own anxiety down and increase their own level of control by taking accountability, but anyone else involved in the situation will also feel their anxiety decrease and sense of control increase.

Another example of when we are able to get control back over our anxiety in a vulnerable situation is when we are pulled over by a police officer while driving. When we see the flashing lights behind us, our anxiety immediately starts to go up. We become nervous, and our thoughts automatically start firing, assuming one thing after another, and very quickly, we are anticipating the worst-case scenario. This is another example of how quickly and easily our automatic thoughts trigger our anxiety and take complete control over our mind. We have a very difficult time focusing on what is happening in the moment. Instead, our anxiety takes over, and we struggle to think clearly, even though we have no evidence that our assumptions are absolutely true or definitely going to happen.

Because we struggle to focus in those moments, we automatically go into defense mode when questioned about why we were driving too fast. Oftentimes, that defense mechanism is presented in the form of justification, giving an excuse as to why we were driving so fast or placing blame on others, such as "Well, the person in front of me was driving the same speed. I was just following him. Why was I the one to get pulled over? Why wasn't the other guy pulled over?"

When we become defensive, our anxiety not only affects us, but it also affects those with whom we are interacting. If a police officer questions us about why we were speeding and all they hear in response are excuses and justification for our actions, they are likely going to react to those defenses by getting annoyed, frustrated, or angry because we are not taking accountability for our actions. When we are making excuses for our behavior, our anxiety may come down slightly on the scale, just for a moment, because in that moment, we are convincing ourselves that what we have done is okay. If we can convince ourselves that what we have done is okay, then we will feel better. This is a false sense of control. Our anxiety is going to quickly return to a higher level on the scale as we are not exercising appropriate control.

In order to actually bring our level of control up, we need to take accountability for our actions. We need to take ownership of the fact that what we choose to do is not right. When we take accountability for our actions, our anxiety will start to decrease, even if we are not sure of the outcome. However, if we choose not to take accountability for our actions, we can easily get into a power struggle with the police officer, and they will likely continue to move forward with giving us a ticket and making sure that we are held accountable for our actions. If we don't hold ourselves accountable for our actions, someone else will.

Accountability and Addiction

Another example of taking accountability is when someone who have been battling addiction acknowledges that they don't have control over their addictive behavior. There is a reason the first step in battling addiction is to admit that there is a problem. That's because when we admit that we have a problem, we are taking accountability. Without accountability, we are limiting ourselves in being able to do the work that needs to be done to get control over the addiction. Although acknowledging there is a problem with addiction is a first step in its treatment, it typically takes awhile for someone to fully understand the breadth of accountability. There is a lot of work involved before someone with an addiction is able to take accountability in all aspects of their life. When someone battling addiction gets to the point where they can fully accept ownership of their actions and choices across all aspects of their life, that is where they make the shift from sobriety to working their recovery. We have to constantly hold ourselves accountable for our behaviors and choices.

This is not only with regard to our addictive behaviors but any behavior or choice in any life domain. If we're only choosing to take accountability sometimes, we're not being honest with ourselves, and we're likely to relapse into maladaptive behavior. We then have to recognize that that is our choice and no one else's. We can't justify our actions and still increase our sense of control over the situation. We have to take 100 percent accountability for and ownership of our choices. Once someone battling addiction is able to take accountability for their choices and own their addiction, they will actually increase their awareness and level of control over their addiction. They know that they are now taking the right steps to get control over their addiction. Again, they can't undo what's been done, but they can shift their focus to what they can do moving forward.

Working with an addiction can be tricky when learning to take accountability. Manipulation is often a survival mechanism for someone with an addiction. I use the word *survival* because someone with an addiction will use whatever means necessary to get what they want or need. The addiction fine-tunes an individual to manipulate others or situations in order to get what they think they need. It is difficult to train the brain to think otherwise and to take accountability for their behaviors when their brain has been programmed to this survival mode to get their substance of choice and prevent them from getting sick.

How Defenses Interfere with Accountability

One reason we often struggle to take accountability is because we don't want to admit when we are wrong, when we make a mistake, when we make a bad decision, or when we flat-out don't have control over something. Unfortunately, we oftentimes interpret these actions as weak and don't want to admit that we are vulnerable. People often make the assumption that something is wrong with us when we are vulnerable. This is a huge misunderstanding. When we take ownership of our actions, we are acknowledging our vulnerability. This is a significant strength. Not only do others have respect for us when we take accountability, but we are increasing our sense of control by addressing our mistakes and vulnerabilities. We are not hiding what we've done but are able to shift our focus to what we can do to manage the situation as best we can. We want to focus on the fact that we are doing the right thing by taking accountability and stay focused on our own responsibilities moving forward.

Respect

There is also the matter of the respect that is given to a person who demonstrates accountability. When a person takes responsibility for their actions, others are likely to respect them for it. Continuing with the example of getting pulled over by a police officer, there is a good chance the officer is going to respect you for taking ownership of your driving behaviors. They are also going to feel less frustrated or anxious if they don't feel they are in a power struggle with you. The officer will be more willing to work with you and may even let you off with a warning rather than handing out a ticket if they see that you understand what you did wrong, accept responsibility, and don't fight it.

Another example is if your supervisor recognizes a mistake you made at work. When they address the issue with you, your anxiety is likely to increase in that moment. You may start to assume that your supervisor is going to reprimand you or even that you may lose your job. However, there is no concrete evidence that either of those assumptions is definitely going to happen. Your supervisor would like to see how you handle this situation. Are you willing to acknowledge and take accountability for the mistake, or are you going to justify or give an excuse as to why you did what you did? If you choose to take accountability for your actions, your supervisor is more likely to respect how you handle the situation and not feel the need to continue addressing what you have done wrong. They will be pleased with the fact that you do not give them any excuses, blame anyone else, or justify your actions. Their level of concern will decrease, and they will feel a greater sense of control when handling the situation. They may initially have felt uncomfortable bringing up a delicate situation with you or correcting you and likely do not want to make you feel bad. If you address the situation appropriately, they are likely to feel more comfortable discussing difficult issues in the future, knowing that you are capable of listening to them, communicating effectively, and taking accountability when needed. In addition, you will feel your anxiety decrease, knowing that you have made the right choice to take accountability.

When working with someone who battles addiction, those who are involved in that person's life will also feel great respect when their loved one has worked their way into recovery after learning to fully take ownership of all the choices they have made during their active addiction. They will also see how their loved one continues to take accountability for their choices and actions in the future. This refers to all aspects of life, including relationships, work, self-care, daily responsibilities, etc.

This summarizes what happens to our anxiety when we do and do not take accountability for our actions:

- We may alleviate our anxiety in the moment when we are justifying our behaviors or manipulating others; however, this is only a false sense of control. Our anxiety will drop briefly on the scale but will quickly return to a higher level if we are not acknowledging our role in that situation. We need to be honest with ourselves as well as others if we expect to gain adequate control and bring our anxiety down. By taking accountability for our actions, we know we are doing the right thing, we are not making excuses or justifying our behaviors, we are being honest, and we are not manipulating the situation to our benefit. We are simply acknowledging our role or the choice that we made, which allows us to shift our focus to what we need to do moving forward to improve the situation or prevent it from happening again. Furthermore, when we take accountability for our actions, others are more likely to respect us for taking ownership of making a mistake.
- Others will be less likely to feel anxiety toward us (frustration, annoyance, or anger) for making a mistake if we are able to take full responsibility. When we don't take responsibility for our actions, others often feel frustration toward us, which makes the dynamic more volatile, possibly leading to a power struggle. Person A may point out what person B does; person B becomes defensive and justifies their behavior or choice, leading to person A becoming more

145

frustrated and defensive while continuing to express what person B does that is wrong, while person B is now reactive and talking over person A, so person A raises their voice, and each person is fighting to have control or the upper hand in the situation. Neither person feels like they are being heard. Person B may be feeling attacked, which makes it difficult for them to take accountability for their actions. All these result in a power struggle where neither person feels they have control or have been heard or respected.

Enabling

When we (and kids) are not taught how to take accountability for our actions or understand the importance of it, we struggle to accept when things don't go our way or when we don't get what we want. Kids are going to engage in various behaviors when they don't get what they want upon initial request (or demand). As kids are learning how to navigate their environment, they become master manipulators. This is actually their job when they are toddlers and in latency (between six and twelve years of age). They are trying to figure out what they can get away with and what they can't. This is why it is critical for us as adults to make sure that we are teaching our kids accountability, acceptance when they don't get their way, importance of the word *no*, and ways they can communicate in order to get their needs met more effectively while exercising control in appropriate and healthy ways.

When our kids ask us for something and our response to them is no, they will likely escalate the situation (especially when they are younger) and start to plead or beg for what they want. When the answer is still no, they may continue to up the ante and whine, present a negative attitude, cry, or have a meltdown. Although it is often hard to manage these behaviors, we need to be aware that we are not to enable our kids. If our kids keep up these behaviors and we ultimately give them what they want because we just can't stand listening to the whining or meltdowns, we are giving them what they want. They just learn that if they keep increasing their behaviors, they can manipulate us (or in their minds, trick us) into giving them what they want. The next time they want something and don't get it right away, they know they can eventually break us and get what they want. By giving them what they want, we are enabling them. We aren't teaching them that they have to accept no as an answer sometimes. They aren't learning that they don't always get their way or that things don't always go as planned. We aren't teaching them how to accept that they don't have control over everything or everyone. We aren't teaching them to identify what else they can do in the moment or to find another time when they may be able to do what they want. We are not teaching them how to problem solve on their own. We are enabling them. This is why it is so critical for parents and caregivers to be consistent in setting limits and following through with them.

Let's think about what enabling looks like for someone battling addiction (young adult or older) and living at home with their parents. When parents first learn about their child's addiction, their instinct is to help their child in any way they can, which is understandable. Any parent will hate to see their child struggling with an addiction. It's natural to automatically think about how you can help your child and want to do whatever it takes. However, this is a slippery slope. The child who has the addiction is responsible for themselves and their own treatment. Parents may be able to financially support their child's treatment, but if the child does not take accountability in doing the work to get control over their addiction, they end up being enabled if they know that their parents will continue to pay for their treatment and still provide them with a place to live, food, and financial support, particularly if the child continues to use. Although it is very difficult, it is important for parents to be firm and consistent in setting limits with their child and holding them accountable for their addiction and other harmful or risky choices. Parents can still support their child through communicating, listening, and asking questions about what they are doing to take care of themselves, but it's critical to set firm boundaries between the parents and child.

Resilience

Resilience is a very important aspect of overcoming anxiety and life-altering events, traumatic or otherwise. According to the American Psychological Association (APA), *resilience* is the process of adapting well in the face of adversity, trauma, tragedy, threats, or significant sources of stress and overcoming difficult life experiences. In other words, using control theory, *resilience* is identifying ways in which we can exercise or gain back control in areas of our lives that have been altered or traumatized. This involves processing various emotions, understanding the thought process behind the traumatic experience, and understanding where we feel a loss of control.

The APA lists a number of factors that are associated with resilience. One important factor is the ability to make realistic plans. This is consistent with the idea in control theory of identifying what is within our control and focusing on what we can do to help manage the stressful situation moving forward. This is where we focus on solutions. By identifying possible options to help in a stressful or potentially stressful situation, we are already focusing on what is within our control. Therefore, our sense of control starts to immediately increase. Again, when our sense of control increases, our anxiety simultaneously decreases. Furthermore, by identifying more than one option to manage a stressor, we are utilizing flexibility in thinking. As previously discussed, flexibility in thinking allows us to modify our plans or options according to the situation. When we think too rigidly, we are vulnerable to experiencing higher levels of stress when our only plan does not go accordingly. We can be easily caught off guard and not know what to do if things don't go according to plan when we have such rigid thinking. It is very difficult to think about other possibilities. Flexibility in thinking also helps us accept things over which we don't have control and allows us to shift our focus to what we can do given the circumstances in which we find ourselves, helping us identify what is actually within our control.

This taps into another point that neuropsychologist Dr. William Stixrud (Stixrud and Johnson 2018) addresses in understanding the physiology of the brain when experiencing chronic stress. The hippocampus, which plays an important part in memory, also aids in bringing perspective when assessing stressful situations. The hippocampus draws on memories from past experiences and information that we already learned and puts our current stressful situation into context, helping facilitate our problem-solving abilities. We are able to draw on what possible solutions may work in a given situation and what we know hasn't worked before. We can deduct from previous experiences or what we've learned from others, apply that information to our current situation, and identify possible options to help manage our current stressor.

Stress hormones can help us remember important information so that we are able to recall dangerous situations to avoid them in the future. The hormones help provide a natural defense mechanism and help prepare us to better manage the potential stressor if it happens again. The parts of the brain responsible for learning and memory are also the ones with the most stress hormones (Stixrud and Johnson 2018; Center for Studies on Human Stress 2017). These are the areas that receive the most information about a stressor. When too many or too few stress hormones are activated, our memory is affected.

According to the Center for Studies on Human Stress (CSHS), high levels of stress interfere with our ability to learn new information and to accurately encode, interpret, or recall information. This is one reason students may draw a blank when taking a test, even though they understand the material. Because students are often juggling many responsibilities and are under high stress, their ability to learn new information or recall learned information can be limited.

The prefrontal cortex, hippocampus, and amygdala are critical in learning, memory, and stress management. The prefrontal cortex evaluates the stressful situation to help us make decisions about what to do. The hippocampus is responsible for spatial memory, helping us identify or recall where we encounter a stressor. The amygdala is responsible for our emotional memory, such as fear or threats. All these areas play critical roles in helping us navigate anxiety-provoking life experiences. By identifying information about the stressor, we are then able to utilize our problem-solving skills to shift our sense of control back into our own hands. However, when we experience chronic stress, which results from repeated exposure to stressors that lead to the release of hormones, it causes wear and tear on the mind and body (Stixrud and Johnson 2018). We have a more difficult time recovering from repeated exposure to stressors and processing important information or memories to help us manage the stressors as effectively as we should.

As Dr. Stixrud addresses, acute or short-term stress is an important factor in resilience. Acute stress, according to Dr. Stixrud, occurs during events or situations that include novelty, unpredictability, or threatening to our sense of self and leave us with a poor sense of control. Short-term or intermittent anxiety allows us to recover from the high level of anxiety we experience during that event and use it in a productive way. Acute stress can be helpful because we are able to more quickly learn from these experiences, and the hormones that are released help us manage the situation. This is different from chronic, ongoing anxiety, from which it is more difficult to recover.

Other important factors associated with resilience, according to the APA, are communicating and problem-solving. This is also consistent with control theory, as we emphasize the importance of communication. As previously discussed, communication is one of the biggest tools in exercising control in a healthy and effective way. It's a way in which we can express our emotions, process our thoughts (vocalize any assumptions or anticipatory thoughts and have others clarify information that may have led to those thoughts), set boundaries with others (where we are essentially letting others know that we are in control of ourselves, not anyone else, and don't allow others to manipulate or project their own anxiety onto us), and hold others accountable for their own responsibilities rather than allow others to place their responsibilities on us.

Problem-solving is key to control theory and stems from cognitive theory. In control theory, we work to focus on what is within our control at the present moment and identify what our options are moving forward. Solution-focused therapy is one treatment objective that we use with control theory to identify specific steps in helping manage a stressful situation or circumstance. The objective is to help an overwhelming, high-anxiety situation become more manageable.

By identifying options that are at our disposal or within our control to manage a potentially stressful situation as best we can, we are automatically increasing our sense of control.

We are also utilizing flexibility in thinking, so we are able to identify other options if things don't go as planned. By exercising flexibility in thinking and focusing on other options that are within our control, while accepting what is not within our control, we are preventing ourselves from thinking rigidly. If our plan does not go the way we predict, we don't feel we lose complete control because we have other options. This is what the solution-focused treatment objectives address. By coming up with a plan of how to manage a potentially stressful situation, we are going to feel more prepared if the situation actually materializes. We will have already thought through our options and identified what is within our control. We are more prepared. This preparation in and of itself increases our sense of control immediately, which also decreases our anxiety. Once we identify a plan, we put that plan aside and then focus on what we need to do in the moment. Again, we don't have proof that what we're anticipating will definitely happen, and if it's not currently happening, we want to put our plan aside and shift our focus to what we need to do in the moment.

Self-confidence is another factor the APA lists as being associated with resilience. This is also consistent with control theory when applying a scale from 0 to 10, where self-confidence goes hand in hand with our sense of control. As previously discussed, if we feel competent in certain areas of our lives or know that we have certain strengths and skills, we are going to feel a greater sense of control. Thus, when we feel we have more control, we are more confident that we will be equipped to manage stressors that arise in the future. If we know what we're capable of doing, we can better predict what we can do to manage a stressful situation. When situations are more predictable, we're going to feel a greater sense of control and, therefore, a lower level of anxiety.

Taking Care of Ourselves

Self-care is critical in helping manage anxiety. There are some important factors that play a direct role in how anxious we may feel on a daily basis. One of the main factors that highly influence our anxiety is sleep. As previously discussed, when we don't get the amount of sleep that we need or the quality of sleep that we need, we are automatically more vulnerable to developing higher levels of anxiety. We have a harder time focusing or concentrating; we are more irritable, have less patience, and are more likely to react quickly and negatively in stressful situations.

Some of the basic self-care objectives that we are able to have greater control over include eating healthy food; making sure that we eat something for breakfast to help improve our cognitive functioning; creating a consistent sleep-wake routine; limiting our intake of caffeine, alcohol, and alternate substances; and incorporating physical exercise. Exercising does not need to be extreme; even a ten-minute walk every day, for example, can help.

I recommend limiting caffeine intake, especially in the afternoon. I typically recommend not having any caffeine after noon, as the caffeine stays in our system for up to twelve hours. If we have a cup of coffee at 4:00 p.m., the caffeine will still be at half its strength six hours later when we are trying to fall asleep, therefore, interfering with getting the deep, restful sleep that we need.

Eating breakfast is also critical in helping us manage our anxiety more effectively. When we don't get the nutrients we need, especially after several hours of fasting overnight, we have a harder time focusing, concentrating, and managing stressors as effectively as we should. These are things that we can choose to implement into our daily routines that help facilitate our ability to perform better across domains as well as helping us manage our anxiety more effectively.

Understanding Relapse

What does it mean to relapse? Relapsing is reengaging in maladaptive behavior, usually in a time of high stress. Relapse can happen after we start working on abstaining from engaging in our maladaptive behaviors for any period of time.

We are all vulnerable to relapse when we are experiencing a high level of anxiety. Relapse can happen when we are having a difficult time identifying our automatic thoughts or the source of the anxiety and have been struggling to focus on ourselves and what our responsibilities are in the moment. We are particularly vulnerable to relapse when we struggle to take accountability for our actions and choices. It is critical to understand the importance of this responsibility we have to ourselves.

Let's recall what can easily happen when our anxiety is at the top of the scale, and we are feeling entirely overwhelmed. When we are completely consumed by our anxiety, the easiest thing for us to do in the moment is engage in whatever is at our fingertips, whether it be blaming others, substance use, self-harm, or any other type of avoidance. Avoidance is the easiest defense mechanism to help alleviate our anxiety. Unfortunately, it is much easier to engage in the old maladaptive behaviors we are so used to or conditioned to. It takes more work, mentally, emotionally, and cognitively, to take the appropriate steps to decrease our anxiety in a healthy way. It takes work to resist the impulses that can bring us temporary relief so quickly, often immediately.

When we are experiencing such a high level of anxiety that it is consuming us, we are not able to think clearly or focus on what we are in control of in the moment. This is why it is critical for us to learn how to use cognitive objectives as a preventive measure so we don't continue to engage in the maladaptive behaviors we are so used to in a time of high stress or crisis. It takes constant practice to become more aware of anxiety, understand how we perceive and interpret information, be able to identify our automatic thoughts, recognize what thoughts are valid or not, identify what our options are when experiencing high anxiety (problem solve), shift our focus to what we are doing in the moment, and identify what is within our control. It takes continuous practice to shift our focus from what others are doing around us or trying to meet others' expectations to what we need to be doing for ourselves and what is in our own best interests. We are essentially reconditioning our brain to think differently than it's been doing our entire lives. This takes time. However, as we practice these objectives, we will be decreasing the likelihood of a relapse as well as the duration, intensity, and frequency of symptoms caused by anxiety, including depression. By increasing our level of control over our anxiety, we will be increasing our level of control across all areas of our lives.

Medications

Let's review what we have discussed about defense mechanisms and substance use. If we are high on the scale and don't have the awareness or the clinical tools to help manage and appropriately control our anxiety, we often use whatever is at our fingertips to help alleviate that awful feeling of being at an 8, 9, or 10 on the scale. There are numerous behaviors in which we can engage to help alleviate that terror as we've previously discussed. These maladaptive behaviors can help us feel better in the moment so we don't have to do the work to reflect on what our responsibility is to ourselves or what the steps are to appropriately and healthily manage our anxiety or depression.

However, these options will only bring temporary relief. Our anxiety is going to go right back up on the scale. These behaviors will give us a false sense of control. Medication will serve the same purpose of helping us feel better. However, medication does not take away the source of anxiety and doesn't teach us how to manage the anxiety ourselves when not used in conjunction with therapy. Just like any other substance, we can eventually become dependent on the medication to help us feel better rather than depending on our problem-solving skills to get control over the anxiety.

Over time, we build up a tolerance to the medication. As a result, the dose of the medication is increased, or another medication is added to the prescription to help manage the symptoms. Ultimately, many people end up having their medications continuously increased, whether by the dose or by adding supplemental medications or having to go through medication changes. This can cause side effects, which can be detrimental or create additional stressors to our daily functioning. When is this pattern going to end if we aren't taught how to actively manage our anxiety? Who wants to be dependent on medication for the rest of their lives for something that can be healthily and naturally controlled? Let's at least minimize the amount of medication we are on if necessary and work on building up our own sense of control and self-confidence in being able to tackle anxiety and know that we are capable of taking care of ourselves.

Again, if there is any progress in our clinical work (becoming more aware of our baseline level of anxiety, understanding our thought patterns and our interpretation of information or situations, or identifying what we are able to do to manage a stressful situation as best we can), resulting in even a slight decrease in anxiety, then there is evidence that we are depending on our own skills to help manage our anxiety. Let's not assume that medication is a necessity from the starting gate.

PART 4

Control Theory in Practice

Understanding the Importance of Mental Health Education in Schools: Preventing Tragedies

Approximately one in five students suffer from some symptom of mental illness (American Psychiatric Association 2016). Anxiety disorders are the most common mental health illness in the United States, affecting forty million adults ages eighteen and older, which is 18 percent of the population (Anxiety and Depression Association of America 2015). Only one-third of those suffering receive treatment. Anxiety affects one in eight children (at a clinical level), and when not treated, students are at higher risk for poor school performance, increased maladaptive and risky behaviors, and increased interference with social functioning (CDC 2018).

Schools can serve as crucial facilitators in aiding students with education on what mental health is, particularly with regard to helping students understand anxiety and the role it plays in their lives. Unfortunately, the US education system is more achievement oriented than child oriented. Children need to be empowered to live effectively in the world, independent of their academic achievements. Empowered children will be more resilient and will be able to utilize control in ways that are not maladaptive but more solution focused.

Teaching students objectives such as anxiety management, stress tolerance, emotional regulation, interpersonal skills, and solution-focused work can help prevent them from developing more severe mental health issues or engaging in other maladaptive behaviors. They can utilize these same tools across domains, whether it's managing academics, being at home, being in social situations, being peer pressured, bullying, using substances, or having body image issues, and, of course, these can help them exercise control over their general anxiety. The result will be as follows:

- Increased self-esteem or self-confidence
- Increased sense of self
- Increased ability to manage stress
- Stronger problem-solving skills
- More learning to take accountability for their choices, actions, and behaviors
- Increased focus on themselves and their own responsibilities rather than focusing on others or comparing themselves to others
- Increased interpersonal/communication skills, leading to more positive, healthy relationships
- Increased school attendance

By learning how to exercise more control over their anxiety, they will be less likely to use substances to alleviate their anxiety, therefore, helping prevent substance use and dependence. Controlling anxiety can aid in preventing or minimizing self-injurious behaviors, including cutting or behaviors that can lead to eating disorders. Knowing how to control anxiety can prevent or decrease the likelihood that students will be bullied or even act as bullies. Students will learn ways to take accountability and understand how they gain more control from taking responsibility for their choices. They will be able to focus on themselves more instead of focusing on what they think others want them to do or comparing themselves to others.

There is clearly a lack of preventive services within school systems. Students need education about mental health before they start to experience severe depression or other mental health issues. It is not enough to help provide support after something extreme happens to an individual student or an entire school. We need to teach students what they can do to take care of themselves before they get to a point of hopelessness or find themselves too deep in a pattern of unhealthy behaviors.

Furthermore, by educating students about anxiety and mental health, we can normalize mental health and anxiety. If schools really want to destigmatize mental health issues, it's not enough just to refer students to mental health-care providers after they have been experiencing extreme anxiety or depression for a prolonged period of time. We need to normalize anxiety. We can help them understand that every single person has anxiety, yet it does not mean that they have a disorder. We want students to understand that nothing is wrong with them if they are feeling anxious, but we want them to have more awareness about their own anxiety. Additionally, if a student continues to feel overwhelmed with anxiety and depression, we want them to recognize that they may need additional help and feel that it is okay to reach out for that help. Again, it does not mean that something is wrong with them. Anxiety plays a significant role in our daily lives, and it cannot be emphasized enough that students need to learn what anxiety is and how they can best control it.

Another reason for providing this type of education in schools is that school counselors are overloaded. It is nearly impossible for counselors to provide individual time for all the students who feel they need help. It is also common for students not to recognize when they are overwhelmed with anxiety until their lives start to feel unmanageable, and they may be embarrassed to ask for help. By providing an educational forum for students, we can provide them with a level of insight so they become aware of their anxiety and can start to utilize tools to get control over it. There are too many students who are in need of services and who are not receiving them or the support they need due to the ratio of students to counselors.

Not only is it overwhelming for school counselors and those students who want to be seen, but it can be a burden on the students and families if they are trying to access care outside of the school. Health insurance may not be required to cover mental health treatment down the road, therefore, limiting students' (or anyone's, for that matter) access to mental health services in their community. To further complicate the accessibility of mental health services, there are more and more providers practicing out of network with insurance companies, which again limits provider availability when most families are not able to pay out of pocket for these services. If students (and parents) are provided with an educational base on anxiety and mental health, we can help facilitate their getting basic help in managing anxiety to inoculate them against falling victim to stressors. It provides an opportunity for students and families to learn how to communicate with each other and how to create a dialogue within their families or with the school about a student's struggles.

Another critical factor that mental health education can work to prevent or decrease is the likelihood of school refusal. There is a new federal education law, Every Student Succeeds Act (ESSA), which requires schools to measure their success using five particular measures. Four of those measures are strictly based on academic performance, but the law allows the fifth measurement to be decided by the states. At this time, the majority of states are choosing to measure school success by measuring "chronic student absenteeism" (NPR 2017), which is the most popular nonacademic measurement of school success. However, absenteeism is measured using a statistical measure and not by understanding why students are absent or what prevents them from attending class. Research tends to focus on the prognosis of students who are not attending school not necessarily what precipitates a student's decision not to attend. Research suggests that students who are chronically absent are more likely to fall behind in school and drop out completely (Young 2017). The most recent studies of school absentee rates found that more than six million students are "chronically absent," meaning absent more than 10 percent of the total number of days for the school year (NPR 2017).

Even though there are studies that track the rate of student absenteeism, there are no concrete action plans to address or decrease student absentee rates, other than giving consequences for offenders. Giving students consequences for not attending school is not going to help the students feel supported, understood, or more motivated to attend school and for the right reasons. Nor will these consequences help students feel like they are provided an opportunity to address what is preventing them from attending school. Consequences can actually be more of a deterrent for students than a way of getting them to attend school. In order for schools to improve their students' success rate, they need to understand what factors prevent students from attending school, provide support for students and their families, and understand why it can be difficult for their students to attend school.

Schools need to identify factors that contribute to students not attending school. Are they being bullied, having a hard time separating from their parents, feeling afraid of being judged, or having other negative experiences at school? All these situations present dynamics in which a student's sense of control is minimized. Schools need to be aware of the fact that, when students do not feel they have adequate control in certain areas of their lives, they are at an increased risk of missing school. Their anxiety, related to school or not, is likely to be contributing to school avoidance or other maladaptive behaviors.

One other benefit that mental health education in schools can provide is a preventive measure for school violence. We are continuously witnessing acts of violence in schools, especially over the past couple of decades, which seem to be increasing in frequency. By teaching students ways in which they can gain healthy control back in their lives and exercise control in appropriate ways (rather than using control in maladaptive ways), we can help prevent violence. Violence is yet another way in which control is exercised wrongly, which is rooted in anxiety and not having an adequate sense of steering the course of one's life. We need to help our students understand their anxiety and where it comes from and help them gain back healthy control in their lives before hurting the lives of others. Those who engage in violent behavior are not likely to know any other way to successfully manage their anxiety and mental health. Control is the key factor that drives their behavior. Wouldn't you want someone who has access to firearms to have other means of controlling their anxiety and anger, helping prevent them from engaging in violence? I would.

Because mental health is such a significant and broad topic, it's important for students to understand the role anxiety plays in their everyday lives, as well as in their own family dynamics. Whether students come from strained family dynamics, experience extreme anxiety due to academic or social expectations, are being bullied in school, have experienced stressful or abusive relationships, or have a history of trauma, we can help them learn ways to manage these situations, to focus on their needs, and to identify factors over which they have control. Students are more likely to be successful in school when they feel they have more control in other aspects of their lives. This does not necessarily mean changing the circumstances that are causing such stress for students but teaching them how to identify and focus on factors over which they do have control. We can help them identify options (focusing on solutions) that are more manageable and realistic in exercising control in their stressful environments.

According to the WHO, there is very little financial investment for mental health services. Even in high-income countries like the United States, nearly 50 percent of people suffering from depression are not receiving the help that they need. For every dollar invested in mental health treatment, specifically for anxiety and depression, according to the WHO, there is a return of four dollars (US) in better health and ability to work. In our current state of health care and insurance, insurance companies are required to cover costs for mental health and substance use treatment. However, insurance companies are paying the providers less and less, while subscribers are paying more and more for their coverage and getting minimal benefits. Providers have a hard time keeping up with the cut in their contracted rates and are increasingly discontinuing their participation with insurance panels, which leaves subscribers having to pay more out of pocket for their treatment. This system is critically flawed. Again, this highlights the need for mental health education and preventive work to be provided in the schools so families won't be stuck having to pay excruciating amounts of money for basic mental health education and support for their children. Also, when people are not able to get the help they need, they oftentimes find themselves struggling to attend school or work, which puts a financial burden on families when a parent is not able to work, either for mental health reasons or because they are taking care of a child who is not able to go to school.

Lastly, Florida recently enacted a law that requires students to provide information on whether they have been referred for mental health services upon registering for school. This is in an effort to identify at-risk students and was prompted after the mass shooting of seventeen students at Marjory Stoneman Douglas High School in February 2018. Four hundred million dollars have also been dedicated to providing mental health resources in Florida public schools. With this money, more psychologists and counselors have been hired to help manage mental health concerns in the schools. However, this approach can be more damaging than it is helpful. First, by providing schools with personal mental health information, students and their families will feel more stigmatized than ever, not to mention that this information will be in the students' permanent records. Students and parents are likely not going to want to provide personal information. Second, mental health information is confidential. Regardless of whether there are resources and mental health professionals available, students are going to be more focused on how they are judged and treated than on accessing help at school. They will continue to feel stigmatized if schools don't address mental health appropriately in an educative and preventive way. Because mental health is as stigmatized as it is, those who suffer from mental health issues, even basic anxiety, are likely going to assume that they are in a different classification than their "normal" peers. Acknowledging mental health issues or the need to reach out for help can be, and often is, interpreted as a weakness or that something is wrong with them. I feel this approach to managing mental health issues in the schools is headed in the absolute wrong direction.

Program Success

One of the programs I worked at during my doctoral training was an intensive community-based acute treatment center, the Wetzel Center, in Worcester, Massachusetts. This program was a step-down facility from a hospital, where kids, ranging from ages six to eighteen, were housed and treated when they were discharged from a hospital but were not stable enough to go back into their communities. There were two separate units, one for latency-aged kids (between six and twelve years of age) and an adolescent unit (thirteen through eighteen years of age). During the time I worked there, the Wetzel Center had the lowest recidivism rate for inpatient programs across the state. Other programs, as well as insurance companies, would visit the Wetzel Center to see how they ran their program and to understand why it was more successful than other programs in the state. The state-ran health insurance required hospitals to call the Wetzel Center first when stepping a child down to a lower level of care.

However, as well as the Wetzel Center was doing at this time, I was not yet applying my control theory in my practice. I was practicing cognitive-behavioral theory and structural family theory and using a strength-based approach in my work that I learned from my mentor, Dr. Robert Dingman. Dr. Dingman guided me in my practice with my clients, helping them shift their focus so they were not just recognizing the negative behaviors in which they engaged but also looking at how frequently they could have engaged in a negative or maladaptive behavior and chose not to. It was a strength-based approach in which we worked with clients to shift their focus from the things they had done wrong to recognizing how successful they had been at exercising healthy control in their lives.

Although we used a strength-based approach with the clients and the Wetzel Center was a top treatment center in the state, it was not actively recognized by the clinical or unit staff that control was something that was at the root of all the work being done at the center. For several years after working at the Wetzel Center, I often thought about and questioned why the Wetzel Center was so successful. As I started focusing on the role of control in my clinical work, specifically studying more about anxiety, I recognized this same theme in the work that was done at the Wetzel Center.

First, there was constant communication. Clinical and unit staff would meet each morning to discuss cases, inform the team of upcoming or potential meetings, and discuss how each client on the units was doing. We also discussed any issues that came up and options for how to manage those issues. Everyone had an important role and participated in the discussion. There was also communication between the clinical staff, unit staff, and the clients' caregivers, outside providers, schools, and other community service providers. The unit staff would constantly communicate with others about how the clients were doing, who had a visit, who was able to go off unit, how they were doing with other clients on the unit, and any upcoming transitions for clients.

Furthermore, before clients were discharged, the unit and clinical staff would schedule appointments with outside providers to make sure they would have follow-up support when they transitioned back into the community. There would also be case conferences for each client within the first week of their admittance and every couple of weeks thereafter, as well as a discharge meeting, to keep all caregivers and treatment and community providers informed on how each child was doing and what the treatment or discharge plan would be as the clients continued to make progress in their work. The Wetzel Center functioned optimally in large part because of its high level of communication within the units and between clinical staff, families, and outside providers.

The clinical work within the units was just as critical as the communication needed to run the units. This work was also successful as a result of the communication between the unit staff and the clients. Granted, the first two weeks after the clients were admitted were typically difficult. It was a stressful transition for the clients at any age. It was understandable that a child would need some time to adjust to a new place and program, but let's look at the role in which control, or the lack thereof, plays in this transition.

When a child (or anyone, for that matter) is new to any type of environment, their personal sense of control is going to be low. The reason is that when they don't know what to expect, they won't be able to prepare themselves well to quell their anxiety. Unknown factors such as where they are going, who will be there (especially if there won't be anyone familiar there), who will be in charge, what will be expected of them, where they will be staying, how long they will be staying, and when they will be able to see their family contribute to their lack of a sense of control. When we don't know what to expect, our automatic thoughts start racing, and we start assuming the worst is going to happen. Because of this, when a child is new to the unit at a treatment center, they often have a hard time acclimating to their new environment until they start to recognize a consistent routine, and their daily life becomes more predictable.

The units provided clients with a consistent routine every day. Clients quickly learned when they would have to wake up, when they would eat, when they would be in school, when they would have free time, when they could call their families, when they would have groups, and when they would meet with their clinicians. Their day-to-day life was highly structured. This structure created predictability. The predictability helped them gain a greater sense of control over what they would be doing day-to-day, hour by hour. For kids who came from unstructured homes or homes with limited means, this structure and predictability helped them know that they would be getting food that day and when they would be getting that food. It wasn't a guessing game as to whether they would eat every day. They knew that they would be provided basic necessities, including compassion, support, validation, encouragement, and people who wanted them to feel better and were helping them gain the skills to help themselves.

They were taught accountability. If they started to get frustrated with or to bother other clients, they were told to focus on themselves. They learned that they were not in charge of others and that their job was to focus on their own responsibilities. They learned how to accept what was not within their control. If they made a bad choice on the unit, they were given a consequence of losing a pass off the unit. They were also provided opportunities for restitution after making a bad choice. They learned from these experiences that they were accountable for their own choices, not anyone else. They had to focus on themselves and make the right choices for themselves.

After the first two weeks of a client's stay at the Wetzel Center, their anxiety typically decreased significantly as they knew they were in a safe, structured, and predictable environment. It was actually common for clients not to want to leave the Wetzel Center after having been so successful and having formed such important relationships with each other and the staff. More often than not, these clients had not experienced a healthy friendship or been able to allow themselves to be vulnerable and trust that another adult was going to help take care of them and make sure they had food and a bed to sleep in each night. Many of them didn't know what it was like to have a consistent, structured routine and know that they were going to stay safe each day. When they woke up at the Wetzel Center, they knew they were safe. They felt a sense of control that they hadn't experienced before. It was quite empowering for the clients, as well as for the staff, to watch and see their progress.

Control, with regard to anxiety, was not discussed in any of the work on the unit or within the clinical work, but the Wetzel Center had implemented the necessary and fundamental objectives to help clients gain a healthier sense of control in their lives. There was consistency in the clinical staff, including clinicians, psychiatrists, and directors, as well as the unit staff who were with the clients twenty-four hours a day. Taking all these factors into account, it was not surprising that the Wetzel Center became a leading treatment facility.

Unfortunately, there are numerous facilities that focus on alternative objectives where clients are not learning the necessary skills and awareness of their level of functioning. For example, I've had clients who had previously been diagnosed with eating disorders and have spent time in treatment facilities targeted for eating disorders. The experiences that these clients described were in direct opposition to what they needed in order to exercise control over their disorder or symptoms. Clients are often instructed to make a certain weight before being discharged (needing to be at 80 percent of what their weight should be). The necessity for them to get to a healthy weight can be, and often is, a matter of life and death. However, my clients' clinical progress was not measured. Furthermore, their anxiety was not even discussed in terms of understanding the root cause of their eating disorder.

One client was told to "avoid" thinking about what she was eating and to have her parents control everything she ate. My client was not allowed to eat anything if it did not come from her parents. This approach only increased my client's anxiety as she was instructed to avoid taking responsibility for her disorder. She was not provided appropriate clinical education or treatment objectives to actually get control over her anxiety but was told to give complete control to her parents. This completely enabled the client and puts her responsibilities on her parents, which only led to increased anxiety for both the client and her parents. The client's personal sense of control continued to decrease, increasing anxiety and other symptoms, making her more vulnerable to depression and other, more severe symptoms and destructive thoughts rather than helping her manage her eating disorder.

Now let's take a look at another type of program, Alcoholics Anonymous (AA). Here is a program that, even though not everyone who is battling addiction utilizes it, provides some of the core principles that control theory addresses. The most important objective that AA emphasizes is the need to take accountability. In order to work a healthy recovery (not just be sober but actually work their recovery), members have to acknowledge that they don't have control over their addiction. They need to take accountability for their choices and behaviors. This does not just refer to their addiction. As previously discussed, they need to take accountability in all aspects of their life, including relationships (friendships or other), job responsibilities, personal responsibilities, self-care, and other interpersonal situations. Within their recovery, they need to take responsibility for their behaviors that were influenced by their addiction, such as hurting others, risky or impulsive behaviors, or illegal activity. They need to acknowledge that they are personally responsible for the choices they make and for caring for themselves. They cannot be dependent on anyone else to take care of them. Granted, they utilize various support systems, but they are the ones doing the work, not those in their support systems.

Another aspect of AA that control theory addresses is accepting what is not within our control. Recovery (which, again, is different from sobriety) happens when we accept that we don't have control, not only over our addiction but over endless things, including the people in our lives. We have to accept that we are not always going to get what we want. Things aren't always going to go the way we plan. We can't always manipulate people or circumstances in order to get what we want. Once we accept the things over which we don't have control, we are then able to shift our focus to what we can do and what is within our control.

In the 1970s, psychologist Bruce Alexander (2010) studied the effects of highly addictive drugs on rats. In one setting, rats were confined to solitary steel cages, having no social interaction or playful stimulation of any kind. They were completely isolated. The other setting was a group of rats that were provided with social interaction with other rats and a "rat park" in which they could play on different apparatuses at all times. They also cohabited with the opposite sex. As a result, baby rat pups joined the mix. These rats were not confined.

Each of these settings provided access to highly addictive drugs, including morphine, heroin, cocaine, and amphetamine, using the press of a lever, otherwise known as a Skinner box. The researchers were able to measure that amount of substances consumed by the rats in each setting. The study found that the rats that were completely isolated consumed significantly more drugs than the rats in the rat park. In fact, there was minimal use of drugs by the rats in the rat park. The researchers concluded that these highly addictive substances were not consumed if the rats were able to engage in a social environment where their activity and social interactions were not restricted.

Applying control theory, the rats in the rat park had a higher level of control in their lives than the rats who were in solitary confinement. When there is an increased sense of personal control, anxiety is lower, and there is a decreased likelihood of utilizing other methods (e.g., drugs) to alleviate anxious feelings or increase their sense of control. The rats that had a greater level of control and freedom in their environment were less likely to use the drugs that were readily available to them. (See http://www.brucealexander.com/articles-speeches/rat-park/148-addiction-the-view-from-rat-park/ for more information on the study.)

When we feel controlled by outside factors, including people, circumstances, disconnection from others, isolation, trauma, etc., our personal sense of control drops, which automatically increases our anxiety. As our anxiety increases, we become vulnerable to engaging in maladaptive behaviors to alleviate this anxiety, which provides a false sense of control, if we are not aware of this anxiety or how to manage it appropriately. We need to accept the things and circumstances over which we don't have control and then shift our focus to what we can do that is within our control. Doing so will allow us to shape our own destiny and gain personal fulfillment and meaning in our lives.

Cognitive Behavioral Objectives

Here is a review and an outline of the objectives that are addressed in control theory. These objectives can be applied to a school curriculum focusing on anxiety management and mental health education.[1]

1. Emotional regulation: Here is where we work to increase awareness of emotions; provide education on what anxiety is, how it is manifested, and where it is originally rooted; and understand why or when anxiety is likely to be triggered. When we are able to recognize the thought patterns that trigger anxiety, we increase our level of insight into our thought processes and emotions and are, therefore, better able to recognize ways in which we can control our anxiety as opposed to allowing our anxiety to control our thoughts and behaviors.

2. Interpersonal skills: These focus primarily on communication skills—setting personal boundaries; setting limits with others; focusing on ourselves; taking accountability for our own actions and choices; and being able to hold others accountable for their own behaviors, choices, and anxieties. Communication is one of the most important tools we can utilize to increase our sense of control and effectively help lower another person's anxiety and increase their sense of control if we are communicating appropriately with one

---

[1] These strategies are also applicable for students who have ADHD or autism diagnoses.

another and, more specifically, taking accountability for our actions.

3. Stress tolerance: Stress tolerance helps teach us how to accept what we don't have control over, how to shift our focus to what is within our control, and how to recognize what our priorities are and what we need to be focusing on in the moment. In addition to helping students understand the role of control in anxiety, we address planning, organization, and time-management skills to help students learn how to prioritize their responsibilities and manage their time more effectively, which ultimately is another way in which students learn accountability and responsibility.

4. Solution-focused work: Solution-focused work includes cognitive-based objectives to help students and adults stay focused on themselves while learning to work through stressors or anxieties. It promotes flexibility in thinking (as opposed to maintaining rigid thinking, which increases anxiety), problem-solving, having accountability, having responsibility, and learning ways in which we can exercise healthy and appropriate control in stressful circumstances.

Review of Curriculum Goals Regarding Anxiety Management and Mental Health Education

1. Help students understand what mental health means and help normalize anxiety and other symptoms of our mental health. If schools really want to be stigma-free when it comes to mental health, we need to normalize anxiety and mental health for our students.
2. Increase understanding of the relationship between anxiety, depression, and suicidal ideations.
3. Increase understanding of how anxiety affects behaviors (including maladaptive, self-injurious, manipulative, aggressive, impulsive, and avoidant behaviors) and ways to help decrease or prevent these behaviors.
4. Increase understanding of the relationship between anxiety and substance use and addiction, and how to help decrease or prevent substance use.
5. Increase understanding of the relationship between anxiety and bullying and ways to help decrease or prevent bullying for both the victim and the aggressor.
6. Increase understanding of the relationship between anxiety and school avoidance and ways to help decrease or prevent school avoidance while still holding students (and parents) accountable.
7. Provide ways to communicate with students when anxiety is recognized while still holding them accountable for their

responsibilities and teach students how to communicate effectively with others.

8. Help students understand what is within their control while helping them accept what is not within their control and learn how to focus on themselves and their own responsibilities.

9. Provide students with a supportive environment where they feel more willing to utilize therapy if they feel they need additional support.

Incorporating Our Tools

Let's incorporate what we have discussed in our reading and apply the specific steps to help us exercise the control on which we've been focusing.

1. Identify the stressor or triggering circumstance and level of anxiety.
   - Identify contributing stressful factors.
   - Identify where your anxiety is on a scale of 1 to 10.
   - Take space from the triggering situation if your anxiety is at an 8, 9, or 10 on the scale. Your only job when you are this high on the scale is to engage in something to help you calm yourself, such as going for a walk, listening to music, stepping outside, drawing, doing yoga, or meditating. This does not include using alcohol or other substances.

Once you have come down to a 7 or lower on the scale, continue with the following steps.

2. Identify automatic thoughts.
   - Review thoughts to see if they are valid or not.
   - Identify if there is any evidence that these automatic thoughts are absolutely true or that they are definitely going to happen.
3. Shift your focus to what you are doing in the moment.
   - Identify your priority in the moment.

177

- Identify your responsibility right now.
- Focus on one task at a time.

4. Identify if your automatic thoughts are valid.
   - Identify options for managing the potential stressor as best you can.
   - Identify plan A, plan B, and plan C (problem-solving).
   - Put the plan aside and shift your focus back to what you are doing in the moment.

5. Practice recognizing and accepting what is not within your control.

6. Shift your focus to what is within your control.
   - Identify or review what your options are, given the circumstances.
   - Identify plan A, plan B, and plan C (continue with problem-solving).

7. Communicate.
   - Communicate any assumptions or anticipatory thoughts (automatic thoughts) with those involved or of concern.
   - Validate others' concerns and feelings.
   - Set limits or boundaries with others if needed. (Validation of others before setting limits can be very helpful in deescalating the situation as well.)
   - Hold others accountable for their own actions or choices, not taking on their responsibilities or anxieties.
   - Know that it's okay to tell others that you are not able to help them if you are already feeling overwhelmed by your own responsibilities.
   - Tell others to "focus on yourself" if feeling controlled or overpowered by others. Remember that you are in control of yourself. Others do not have control of you.

- Give choices to others when holding them accountable for their behaviors. Put the responsibility onto them rather than trying to control them or engaging in a power struggle.

8. Focus on yourself.
   - Identify your own responsibilities.
   - Identify your own priorities (not what others want you to prioritize).
   - Make decisions that are in your best interest (not in the interest of others). Your job is not to act in ways to please others and meet their needs, especially in an effort to avoid having others become upset. Your job is to focus on making decisions that are in your own best interest, granted your intention is never to hurt, disrespect, or offend others. However, you need to work on accepting that others may not agree or be happy with your decisions or even have the same opinions, but others also have to accept that they don't have control over everyone else.
   - Validate what others want from you or how they feel, but then set your limits and stay focused on what is in your own best interest.
   - Recognize that you are in control of yourself. Others are not in control of the decisions you make. (There are exceptions here for caregiver-child dynamics, including teacher-child dynamics.)

9. Take accountability for your own choices and behaviors.
   - Know that you are not perfect and are bound to make mistakes or poor choices now and then. The important factor on which to focus is how you handle your mistakes. Do you blame others and justify your behaviors, or do you take accountability for your choices and actions?

10. Recognize mental boundaries for yourself.
   - Focus on the fact that you are not doing anything wrong (especially when setting limits with others even if they don't like it) and that you are following through with your own responsibilities.
   - Know that when you attend to your own responsibilities, you are doing your job.
   - Recognize when your anxiety ends and when the anxiety you may be experiencing is likely someone else's anxiety. Ask yourself, *Is this my responsibility?* Again, focus on what your own responsibilities are and be careful not to take on someone else's responsibilities or anxiety.

11. Practice flexibility in thinking.
   - Break tasks down into smaller parts, breaking the all-or-nothing thinking pattern:
      o Engage in a task for ten to fifteen minutes at a time, then reevaluate how you feel.
      o Study for half an hour, take a break, go back to studying for half an hour, take a break.
      o Accomplish one objective at a time. For example, when struggling to get out of bed in the morning, first focus on getting out of bed and getting to the bathroom. Then reevaluate how you feel. If you need to rest a little more, rest for a little bit and then attempt to get up again. You've already shown yourself that you are capable of accomplishing this. If you feel you are okay, focus on the next task of getting dressed. Then reevaluate how you feel again. These objectives also help with focus and concentration, making tasks more manageable rather than your feeling completely overwhelmed.
   - Utilize time management.
   - Use a daily planner.

- Modify plans as needed when something changes. Identify other times when you can get work done. If you can't do what you were planning to do in the moment, when else can you do it? (This also helps with preventing procrastination.)

12. Reevaluate your anxiety on the scale.
    - Has it decreased after taking these steps?
    - Do you feel an increase in your sense of control? Maybe even a sense of relief? Pride?

13. Do a daily or nightly self-check-in, identifying anything you made progress with that day, any accomplishments, successes, goals met, etc. Examples of accomplishments:
    - Getting out of bed in the morning.
    - Eating.
    - Making it to class or work.
    - Making it to the gym when you had little to no motivation.
    - Going to a doctor's appointment when you really didn't want to.
    - Taking a test that you were dreading.

What Can Parents Do?

- Educate yourself about anxiety.
- Focus on your own anxiety. Most highly anxious kids have highly anxious parents. You need to prioritize your own health and be able to understand and appropriately control your own anxiety in order to help or understand your children's anxiety.
- Communicate with your kids. Open up the line of communication and help teach them that by communicating, they are able to utilize the greatest means of control.
- Validate your child's feelings and concerns. You may not agree with how they feel, but what they experience, whether it's their feelings or how they interpret a situation, is real for them. Don't minimize their experience. You won't want your own experiences to be minimized or disregarded. If you want your children to talk with you and be honest, you have to validate and respect their feelings and experiences.
- Pull back on the level of control as kids get older and more independent. Relinquish some control (where appropriate) so they can exercise more control for themselves. Let your kids make mistakes. Let them fail. Kids will learn more from their failures than if they are micromanaged by parents at ages when they need to be learning how to act and make decisions more independently. Kids have to learn how to accept that they are not going to be 100 percent successful at everything they pursue. That's an unrealistic expectation that should not be put onto our kids. It's okay to fail, and

kids grow from failure when provided guidance and education on how to understand failure and to learn what they can do moving forward (i.e., taking accountability and problem-solving). Kids won't learn to solve problems when they are enabled by being micromanaged beyond what is appropriate for their age and development. As parents, you need to communicate with your children effectively and hold them accountable for their own choices and actions, but you can't try to control their every move. Some questions to think about include the following:

o How do your kids handle a situation in which they fail?
- Do they blame others?
- Do they make excuses?
- Do they justify their actions or decisions?
- Do they take accountability for their own choices?
o How do you handle failure?
o What do you think your kids learn from you?

Talk about choices, risk-taking, and natural consequences. Some risk is okay and sometimes necessary to help kids learn what they are capable of accomplishing while simultaneously understanding their limits. For example, if your child chooses not to do their homework or put effort into their classes, they are then choosing to face the natural consequence of not getting a good grade or potentially failing their classes.

- Don't always tell your child what to do in stressful situations but support them by validating their feelings and facilitate the conversation by asking questions about what they have thought of doing, what they have already tried, who they can talk to, what their options may be, etc. By facilitating the conversation, you are helping them learn and practice their problem-solving skills. You are helping them build up their own personal sense of control as well as their confidence that they will be able to manage future stressors more successfully.

- Teach kids interpersonal skills, such as communicating and setting limits with others. Help them understand that others, their peers in particular, do not have control over them. They are in control of themselves. (There are exceptions when parents are in control of their kids, particularly when they are younger, as well as other adult figures in appropriate circumstances, such as a teacher, school personnel, or a supervisor at a job). Teach your kids that they are in control of the choices they make, whether they be good or bad. It is their independent choice to follow through with their responsibilities across different settings. If they choose to not follow through with these responsibilities, they are choosing the natural consequences of their actions. Those choices are under their control. Even if an adult or authoritative figure is speaking to them inappropriately, they can still set a limit with that person, stating they are willing to speak with the adult, but the adult is not to speak to them disrespectfully.

- Help them understand that they don't have control over everything and not everything is going to go their way.

- Teach them to focus on themselves. Focusing on others takes away their personal sense of control. We tend to shift our control to others by allowing others to maintain our attention, neglecting ourselves, and preventing us from focusing on what our priority is in the moment or what is currently in our best interests. Kids need to focus on the control they have for themselves rather than comparing themselves to their peers or making decisions based on what others want from them or think they should or should not do. Help them strengthen their own sense of self.

- Don't accommodate avoidant behaviors. Don't enable them by doing things for them. For example, don't do their homework for them, don't allow them to skip school when they don't want to go, and don't talk to your high school or college student's teachers for them when the student needs to be communicating with their teachers themselves. Facilitate a dialogue or communication by asking them guided questions to help them think about what they can do. Help them do the problem-solving without doing the work yourself. You can still support your kids while at the same time holding them accountable for their own responsibilities.

- Help them understand the importance of regulating social media, again, emphasizing the importance of focusing on themselves.
- Model appropriate use of phones, iPads, and other devices as parents. Have consistent time away from devices to help teach your kids appropriate boundaries between the virtual and real worlds.
- Teach them about the importance of sleep and help them establish and maintain a consistent sleep-wake cycle.
- Support their need to prioritize sleep over homework. Sleep is critical to helping manage anxiety and depression and should not be neglected in order to get homework done.
- Other sleep tips: keep bedrooms cool, don't exercise within four hours of bedtime, and keep the weekend sleep-ins to no more than sixty minutes of additional rest.
- Teach them accountability. Kids need to learn they are responsible and accountable for their own choices. Do not enable your kids by trying to fix their issues or stressors by taking control of the situation yourself. When kids learn how to take responsibility for themselves, they are increasing their sense of control as well as their self-confidence.
- Know the power of a hug: if you don't know what to say in a given moment when your child is hurting or overwhelmed, give them a hug. You don't need to say a word. Just give your child a hug.

We need to help our kids develop internal motivation by allowing them to exercise more control. Naturally, as parents, we want to make things right for our kids and fix their problems. However, the more of our children's responsibilities we take on as parents, especially as they get older, the less likely our kids will be able to develop their own internal motivation or learn how to exercise control in stressful circumstances. Sometimes we need to allow our kids to fail. We need to help them learn what they can do differently in the future and recognize that their own choices have natural consequences and no one else is to blame. They need to understand the importance of accountability. The more we try to control our kids, the more they will push back and the less willing they will be to hear us as parents and apply what we teach. To reiterate a message by Dr. Stixrud, we need to immunize our children against more potentially damaging mental health issues in the future and to prepare them for happy, healthy, and productive lives.

Acknowledgments

I would like to thank the people who have been an incredible support throughout the process of writing my book as well as helping promote my work in the field. I have been very fortunate to have worked with, known, and interacted with so many influential people who have been a driving force for my work.

I want to thank each and every one of my clients throughout my years of practice for providing insight and helping guide my work in cultivating control theory. I have learned immensely from my clients and continue to do so each day. I hope that each person with whom I have worked has been able to walk away from our sessions with a clearer understanding of their anxiety and to shift healthy control back into their lives. I hope that each of our sessions left you with having had a positive experience.

I would like to thank my husband for his unending support both in my clinical and public work and throughout the process of writing this book. I would also like to thank my sons, Andrew and Carter, for helping me navigate and master my own treatment objectives. I hope you will both see the benefits of our work in the years to come.

I want to say thank you to my professors along the way and, in particular, my mentor, Dr. Robert Dingman. I can't express my gratitude to you for teaching, guiding, and supporting me in my work as I transitioned through different stages of my career. Whenever I start to feel settled in my work, I always remind myself of your words and ask myself, *What's next?* Your words have continued to challenge me every day.

I want to express my gratitude to Emily Bratten for taking time to skillfully review my material and for providing more depth to the messages this book aims to address. Your insight and understanding of this subject have been incredibly valuable.

I would like to thank Dr. William Stixrud for helping guide me in this important subject, for allowing me to use your work as a significant reference, and for your support and guidance in producing my book.

I am grateful for my friends and community supporting my work and pushing to get mental health awareness into our schools. Thank you for being advocates for our children and promoting the need for mental health education in our schools.

Last, but definitely not least, my grandfather, Frank Claybourne, has been a significantly influential hero to me. He has been a pioneer in trying to help adolescents who have been incarcerated receive the treatment they need to help them become successful members of their communities. His advanced thinking paved the way for me to carry out his (and my) vision of providing appropriate treatment and resources for our youth.

References

Alexander, B. K. 2010. "Addiction: The View from the Rat Park." http://www.brucealexander.com/articles-speeches/rat-park/148-addiction-the-view-from-rat-park.

American Psychological Association. 2011. "The Road to Resilience." http://www.apa.org/helpcenter/road-resilience.aspx.

Anxiety and Depression Association of America. 2015. "Facts and Statistics." https://adaa.org/about-adaa/press-room/facts-statistics.

Beck, A. T. 1976. *Cognitive Therapy and the Emotional Disorders.* New York: International Universities Press Inc.

Beck, A. T., F. W. Wright, C. F. Newman, and B. Liese. 1993. *Cognitive Therapy of Substance Abuse.* New York: Guilford Press.

Beck Institute. 2018. "Get Informed." https://beckinstitute.org/get-informed/social-stream.

Beck, J. S. 1995. *Cognitive Behavior Therapy: Basics and Beyond.* New York: Guilford Press.

Breus, M. J. 2017. "Exercise and Its Benefits for Sleep." *Psychology Today*, September 6, 2017. https://www.psychologytoday.com/us/blog/sleep-newzzz/201709/exercise-and-its-benefits-sleep.

Centers for Disease Control and Prevention. 2011–2013. "Welcome to WISQARS." http://cdc.gov/injury/wisqars/index/html.

Centers for Disease Control and Prevention. 2017. "Leading Causes of Death Reports 1981–2017." https://webappa.cdc.gov/sasweb/ncipc/leadcause.html.

Centers for Disease Control and Prevention. 2018. "Key Findings: U.S. Children with Diagnosed Anxiety and Depression."

https://www.cdc.gov//childrensmentalhealth/features/anxiety-and-depression.html.

Centers for Disease Control and Prevention. 2018. "Suicide Rising across the US." https://www.cdc.gov/vitalsigns/suicide.

Diagnostic and Statistical Manual of Mental Disorders, Fifth Edition. Washington, DC: American Psychiatric Publishing, 2016.

EMDR Institute Inc. 2019. "What is EMDR?" https://www.emdr.com/what-is-emdr.

Flora, C. 2017. "The Hardest Word." *Psychology Today*, October 2017, 53–56.

Foxman, P. 2007. *Dancing with Fear: Controlling Stress and Creating a Life Beyond Panic and Anxiety.* Alameda, CA: Hunter House Inc. Publishers.

Green, S. 2018. "Florida Law Requiring Students to Inform School Districts on Mental Health History Is Problematic." *Orlando Sentinel*, August 9, 2018. https://www.orlandosentinel.com/opinion/audience/shannon-green/os-ae-school-districts-mental-health-law-20180809-story.html.

Joelson, R. B. 2017. "Locus of Control: How Do We Determine Our Successes and Failures?" *Psychology Today*, August 2, 2017. https://www.psychologytoday.com/us/blog/moments-matter/201708/locus-control.

Kann, L., S. Kinchen, S. Shanklin, K. H. Flint, J. Hawkins, W. A. Harris, R. Lowry, E. O. Olsen, T. McManus, D. Chyen, L. Whittle, E. Taylor, Z. Demissie, N. Brener, J. Thornton, J. Moore, and S. Zaza. 2013. "Youth Risk Behavior Surveillance: United States, 2013." *Morbidity and Mortality Weekly Report* 67, no. 8: 1–114. https://doi: 10.15585/mmwr.ss6708a1.

Lambert, C. 2005. "Deep into Sleep." *Harvard Magazine*, July–August 2005. https://harvardmagazine.com/2005/07/deep-into-sleep.html.

Linehan, M. M. 1993. *Cognitive-Behavioral Treatment of Borderline Personality Disorder.* New York: The Guilford Press.

Margalit, L. 2016. "What Screen Time Can Really Do to Your Kids' Brains." *Psychology Today*, April 17, 2016. https://www.psychologytoday.com/us/blog/behind-online-behavior/201604/what-screen-time-can-really-do-kids-brains.

McEwen, B., and I. Karatsoreos. 2015. "Sleep Deprivation and Circadian Disruption." *Sleep Medicine Clinics* 10. https://www.researchgate.net/publication/272892924_Sleep_Deprivation_and_Circadian_Disruption.

National Institutes of Mental Health. 2019. "Suicide Is a Leading Cause of Death in the United States." https://www.nimh.nih.gov/health/statistics/suicide.shtml.

National Public Radio. 2017. "A Reformed White Nationalist Speaks Out on Charlottesville." All Things Considered. https://www.npr.org/2017/08/13/543259499/a-reformed-white-nationalist-speaks-out-on-charlottesville.

National Public Radio. 2017. "Most States Plan to Use Student Absences to Measure School Success." How Learning Happens. https://www.npr.org/sections/ed/2017/09/26/550686419/majority-of-states-plan-to-use-chronic-absence-to-measure-schools-success.

National Sleep Foundation. 2017. "Beverages to Avoid to Sleep Soundly While Traveling." https://www.sleepfoundation.org/sleep-topics/beverages-avoid-sleep-soundly-while-traveling.

National Sleep Foundation. 2017. "Children's Stress and Sleep." https://www.sleepfoundation.org/sleep-topics/childrens-stress-sleep.

National Sleep Foundation. 2018. "How Blue Light Affects Kids and Sleep." https://www.sleepfoundation.org/sleep-topics/how-blue-light-affects-kids-sleep.

National Sleep Foundation. 2018. "Teens and Sleep." https://www.sleepfoundation.org/sleep-topics/teens-and-sleep.

Psychology Today. 2017. "Bullying." https://www.psychologytoday.com/basics/bullying.

Roberts Stoler, D. "Restorative Sleep Is Vital to Brain Health." *Psychology Today*, April 6, 2017. https://psychologytoday.com/us/blog/the-resilient-brain/201704/restorative-sleep-is-vital-brain-health.

Scutti, S. "US Suicide Rates Increased More Than 25% Since 1999, CDC Says." *CNN*, June 7, 2018. Last updated June 22, 2018. https://www.cnn.com/2018/06/07/health/suicide-report-cdc/index.html.

Stixrud, W., and N. Johnson. 2018. *The Self-Driven Child: The Science and Sense of Giving Your Kids More Control over Their Lives*. New York: Viking.

Substance Abuse and Mental Health Services Administration. 2014. "Results from 2013 National Survey on Drug Use and Health: Mental Health Findings," NSDUH Series H-49, HHS Publication No. (SMA) 14-4887. Rockville, MD: Substance Abuse and Mental Health Services. https://www.samhsa.gov/data/sites/default/files/NSDUHmhfr2013/NSDUHmhfr2013.pdf.

Twenge, J. 2017. *iGen*. New York: Atria Books.

World Health Organization. 2017. "'Depression: Let's Talk,' Says WHO, as Depression Tops List of Causes of Ill Health." https://www.who.int/en/news-room/detail/30-03-2017--depression-let-s-talk-says-who-as-depression-tops-list-of-causes-of-ill-health.

Yale News. 2008. "Bullying-Suicide Link Explored in New Study by Researchers at Yale." *Yale News*, July 16, 2008. https://news.yale.edu/2008/07/16/bullying-suicide-link-explored-new-study-researchers-yale.

Young, J. L. "Understanding School Refusal: What Parents Need to Know at Back-to-School Time." *Psychology Today*, September 11, 2017. https://www.psychologytoday.com/us/blog/when-your-adult-child-breaks-your-heart/201709/understanding-school-refusal.

About the Author

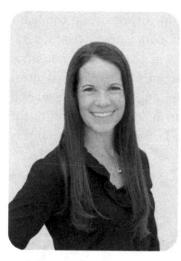

Dr. Jolene Arasz is a practicing psychologist in northern New Jersey. She specializes in anxiety management as it is at the root of any mental health issue. Dr. Arasz currently has a private practice working with adolescents, adults, and families. She received a dual degree in psychobiology from Albright College. From there, she attended the Massachusetts School of Professional Psychology to earn her doctoral degree in clinical psychology. Throughout her doctoral education, she did clinical training in various settings, including outpatient services for adults with major mental illness, elementary and middle school systems, and the Boston Juvenile Court Clinic, and did inpatient and outpatient work with the agency YOU Inc. in Worcester, Massachusetts. She continued her postdoctoral training with YOU Inc., laying the foundation for much of the clinical work she continues today. There, Dr. Arasz worked with children between the ages of six and eighteen, providing intensive individual, group, and family therapy in an inpatient setting. She collaborated with state agencies, families, schools, psychiatrists, and other doctors to facilitate continuous care once the patients were discharged from the program. Since then, she was the clinical director of a substance abuse treatment center for those who were homeless and fighting addiction, as well as providing outpatient services for children, adolescents, and families.

Dr. Arasz now resides in Allendale, New Jersey, with her husband and two remarkable boys. She started her private practice in 2012, where she continues to work with her clients on managing their anxiety and provides an educational approach to her work. She also collaborates with local schools, providing professional development training to teachers and school personnel, and speaks publicly with parents to help them understand anxiety and mental health.

Dr. Arasz is very passionate about her work. She decided to write this book after more than fifteen years of practice in the field, recognizing a major theme throughout her work across settings, ages, demographics, and diagnoses. The theme was anxiety and that anxiety is rooted in lacking a sense of personal control. Dr. Arasz's control theory can be applied to all ages. She is a strong advocate for mental health education becoming a requirement in school curriculum for all ages. This book is aimed at driving the important message of this need.

CPSIA information can be obtained
at www.ICGtesting.com
Printed in the USA
LVHW010155100221
678885LV00003B/424

9 781662 413919